Professional Interpersonal Skills
for Nurses

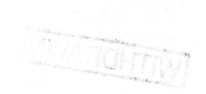

Professional Interpersonal Skills for Nurses

Carolyn Kagan

Lecturer at Manchester Metropolitan University, UK, and works with North Western Training and Development Team, UK

Josie Evans

Huddersfield University, UK and South Manchester Health Authority, UK

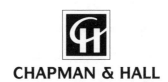

CHAPMAN & HALL

London · Glasgow · Weinheim · New York · Tokyo · Melbourne · Madras

Published by Chapman & Hall, 2-6 Boundary Row, London SE1 8HN, UK

Chapman & Hall, 2-6 Boundary Row, London SE1 8HN, UK

Blackie Academic & Professional, Wester Cleddens Road, Bishopbriggs, Glasgow G64 2NZ, UK

Chapman & Hall GmbH, Pappelallee 3, 69469 Weinheim, Germany

Chapman & Hall USA, One Penn Plaza, 41st Floor, New York NY 10119, USA

Chapman & Hall Japan, ITP - Japan, Kyowa Building, 3F, 2-2-1, Hirakawacho, Chiyoda-ku, Tokyo 102, Japan

Chapman & Hall Australia, Thomas Nelson Australia, 102 Dodds Street, South Melbourne, Victoria 3205, Australia

Chapman & Hall India, R. Seshadri, 32 Second Main Road, CIT East, Madras 600 035, India

First published in 1986 as *A Manual of Interpersonal Skills for Nurses. An experiential approach.*

This edition 1995

© 1995 Carolyn Kagan and Josie Evans

This edition not for sale in North America and Australia; orders from these regions should be referred to Singular Publishing Group, Inc., 4284 41st Street, San Diego, CA92105, USA

Typeset in 10/12pt Palatino by Best-set Typesetter Ltd, Hong Kong
Printed in Great Britain by Page Bros (Norwich) Ltd

ISBN   0 412 44100 4

For Mark

Contents

Contents

Preface

This book is a sequel to an earlier book *A Manual of Interpersonal Skills for Nurses: An Experiential Approach* written by Carolyn Kagan, Josie Evans and Betty Kay in 1986. At that time interpersonal skills was relatively new to nursing curricula, and all nurse basic and post-basic training syllabi contained some aspects of interpersonal skills. Teachers were also new to the area and many were anxious about how they were to introduce experientially based interpersonal skills learning into their courses.

Since that time, nurse education has changed. Project 2000 has been introduced and post-basic training courses have been integrated with higher education. Schools of nursing have combined to form colleges of health in partnership with, or with courses accredited by, institutions of higher education. There has been a shift from experiential exploration of interpersonal skills to the need for an academic understanding of material underpinning interpersonal skill in nursing.

The Health Service, too, has changed. Steadily and unrelentingly throughout the 1980s, health service management and organization has changed. The roles of patients and other consumers of health care have been evolving. Purchaser/provider splits have permeated acute and long-term sectors in hospital, and community and primary care. Trusts have emerged, nurses have been regraded and it is highly unlikely that any nurse is doing the same job, in the same kind of health service, as s/he was doing in 1986. Indeed, in 1994 there is a far greater range of employers of nurses than there was in 1986, with the rapid growth of the independent health care sector.

All of these changes mean that there are new demands being made on nurses in their use of interpersonal skills, and we have incorporated discussion of many of these into this book. So, there are totally new sections on handling pressure, working with groups, managing change, handling conflict, aggression and violence, and supervision, appraisal and performance review. Some sections remain much as they were in the earlier book, as we remain convinced that they form the basis of professional interpersonal skills in nursing. Familiar sections making a reappearance are those focusing on self-awareness; fundamental interpersonal processes (speech, non-verbal behaviour, social perception);

rapport and facilitation; counselling; social problem solving; and constraints on the effective use of interpersonal skills.

Throughout, reference to the parent disciplines of social psychology and to the nursing literature have been incorporated. Details of experiential exercises and their management in the classroom have been omitted – these are still to be found in the 1986 book. Each chapter has some self-development exercises. We think we have made these up; however it is in the nature of interpersonal skills development exercises that sometimes people think particular exercises should have been attributed to them. We apologize if we have omitted to acknowledge anyone's work or ideas.

Two features have been retained but appear in different forms. Illustrations from real nursing situations are clearly marked in boxes. These include illustrations from a far wider range of nursing situations, including community (district nursing, learning disability and psychiatric nursing, school nursing and practice nursing) and hospital episodes. All the examples we have used have been witnessed directly or indirectly: none of them are fiction. We have also drawn attention to areas of controversy, dealt with inadequately by the literature, but central to nursing practice. Thus, questions are raised in 'Food for Thought' boxes.

We hope the book meets contemporary needs for the continuing development of professional interpersonal skills in nursing.

Since writing the earlier book, we too have undergone change. Carolyn is a social worker who works as a lecturer in social psychology at what is now the Manchester Metropolitan University. Since 1987 she has been seconded to work part-time with the North Western Training and Development Team. This is a small multidisciplinary team of two full-time equivalent people, offering consultancy to health and social services for people with learning disabilities in the North Western Region (19 health districts, 11 social service authorities and an increasing number of health trusts and GP fundholders). She works at the interface of interpersonal and professional development, organizational change and user empowerment. Josie has moved to a joint post with Huddersfield University and South Manchester Health Authority, running a satellite Diploma in Nursing course in the Authority, as part of the professional nursing development programme. She is currently researching the contribution continuing professional development makes to the quality of nursing care, and patients' perceptions of 'comfort'.

Betty Kay, who contributed to the earlier book, has been unable to write this one. Her commitments have meant that she has, regrettably, been unable to continue beyond the initial stages. However, we remain indebted to her for her continued interest, support and sense of humour.

The writing of the book has detracted from family life as, despite exhortations from the Higher Education sector urging staff to publish, few resources are provided to enable books to be produced. So it has been written at weekends and evenings alongside massive increases in our workloads in both universities and in the field.

Carolyn would like to thank Mark Burton, Amy Kagan and Anna Kagan for their tolerance and acceptance that the book did, indeed, have to be finished. Anna deserves special mention for keeping her desk tidy and making it available. It is the only table surface in Carolyn's house that is reliably clear. Amy deserves special mention for the continual supply of herb teas throughout days devoted to writing. Mark deserves special mention for cooking, help with the intricacies of the computer, as well as for listening, even though he too has had writing deadlines to meet – and miss.

Josie would like to thank family and friends for their continuing support and encouragement.

We are grateful for the typing assistance given by Pauline Mook and Pauline Stevens and for the support and friendship of colleagues, especially Sue Lewis and Mildred Austin.

While we have been preparing the manuscript our publishers have changed twice. Lisa Fraley has proved to be a supportive and tolerant editor at Chapman & Hall, as deadline after deadline has been passed. We appreciate the lack of pressure put upon us as we have struggled to meet competing demands from our different strands of work.

Carolyn Kagan and Josie Evans,
1993, Manchester

CHAPTER 1

Introduction

In this introduction we intend to set out key features of our approach to professional interpersonal skills in nursing. We do not propose a literature review of the field (indeed, in many ways the rest of the book provides this) but will clarify those assumptions that underlie our observations and discussions.

Our approach to professional interpersonal skills in nursing is one that goes beyond theories and models of communication or social skills. It is one that is firmly grounded in the social psychology of interpersonal and social behaviour and experience. Furthermore, it takes for granted the interdependence of interpersonal experience, behaviour, role and context. What may be professionally skilled in one interpersonal situation may not be in another. What may be professionally skilled on the part of one nurse may not be on the part of another. The keys to professional interpersonal skills in nursing are flexibility and understanding.

'Interpersonal skills refer to those interpersonal aspects of communication and social skills that people [need to] use in direct person-to-person contact' (Kagan, Evans and Kay, 1986, p. 1). Professional interpersonal skills in nursing refer to those particular interpersonal skills nurses have to employ to be effective practitioners, managers or teachers. These professional interpersonal skills can be used when working with patients, patients' relatives, colleagues, other health and welfare practitioners and students. They may be employed in one-to-one, small group or large group encounters. They are not simply those personal qualities nurses bring to their work and their lives. Instead they are the purposive social acts that nurses display at work, while nursing (in its broadest sense). It is the use of such interpersonal skills in the process of nursing that makes them professional interpersonal skills.

Professional interpersonal skills require flexible adaptation to changing circumstances and different people in a range of different situations, in pursuit of clear nursing goals. A number of assumptions stem from this broad definition and underpin the skills approach to nurses' interpersonal transactions outlined in this book.

- Firstly, professional interpersonal behaviour in nursing is learnt. Nurses bring with them their prior learning (and sometimes mis-learning) of interpersonal skills and develop these as they learn, and become experienced in, nursing.
- Secondly, interpersonal behaviour can be broken down into component parts, each of which can be identified, practised and combined with others to improve overall levels of professional competence in different nursing settings.
- Thirdly, professional interpersonal behaviour is made up of cognitive and emotional components as well as behavioural ones.
- Fourthly, complex interpersonal behaviour is underpinned by fundamental elements which combine in different ways for different professional interpersonal skills.
- Lastly, effective deployment of professional interpersonal behaviour may be weakened or prevented by both internal and external constraints: motivation and ability are necessary but not sufficient preconditions to effective professional interpersonal behaviour.

So, a skills perspective on professional interpersonal skills in nursing encourages a look beyond the personal qualities of individual nurses in order to understand the interpersonal nature of nursing. It is also necessary to understand some of the social psychological processes underpinning interpersonal aspects of nursing in order to know what is required in the development of professional interpersonal skills.

Understanding the self, communication, social cognition attitude formation and change, and group dynamics can all help nurses become more effective in some of the complex interaction settings within which they work.

The essence of nursing is interpersonal contact. Nurses do things for and with other people. To do this effectively they need, therefore, to be interpersonally skilled. They need to have command of fundamental interpersonal skills and be able to combine these to form complex and professional interpersonal skills. While these skills are relevant to all the caring and people-focused professions, nurses do have unique situations in which they must exercise their skills. Professional interpersonal skills are not, then, confined to nurses, but the uses to which they are put in nursing are indeed special.

Kagan, Evans and Kay (1986) argued that there are four levels at which interpersonal skills in nursing should be considered. These levels are illustrated in Figure 1.1.

At the very least, nurses should gain insight into their own interpersonal skills and why they might not be using them as effectively as they could at work. This insight will help them achieve greater flexibility in the use of interpersonal skills. Most nurses will need to develop some specialist skills and extend their existing skills to new

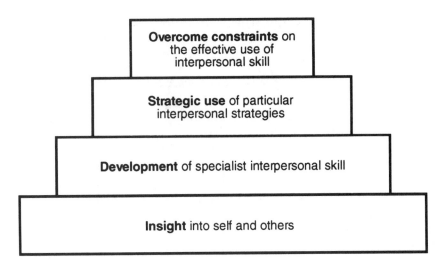

Figure 1.1 Levels of interpersonal skills.

nursing settings. To be able to adapt to new and unpredictable events, nurses must become strategic in their use of specific interpersonal strategies for particular purposes. Finally, nurses need to be able to identify and overcome both internal and external constraints to the effective use of interpersonal skills. The professional use of interpersonal skills requires consideration of all four levels and the return to each level over time. Thus, for example, personal insight is never finished; it may be returned to once specialist skills have been acquired, strategies clarified or constraints overcome.

Nurses will always be able to improve their interpersonal skill, at each level, however skilled they are at any point in time. It is the insight into, evaluation of and ability to change their own interpersonal behaviour that will enable nurses to enhance their professional practice.

There are a number of other assumptions underlying the approach to professional interpersonal skills adopted in this book stemming from Kagan, Evans and Kay (1986).

1. Self-awareness is central to professional interpersonal skill.
2. The understanding, evaluation and change of interpersonal strategies is fundamental to professional interpersonal skill.
3. Some specialist professional interpersonal skills for nursing can be identified and taught.
4. The development of effective professional interpersonal skill is a continuing process, not an end point.
5. Professional interpersonal skills take place in social contexts which may inhibit their effective use.

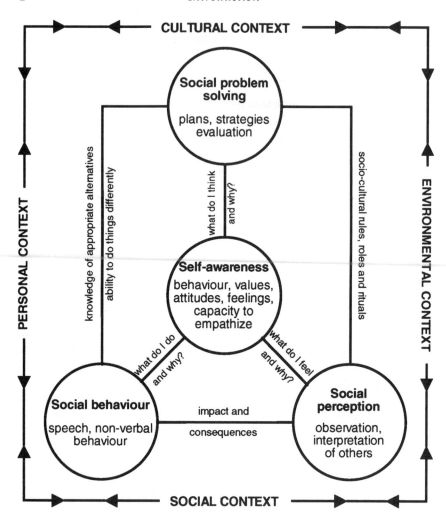

Figure 1.2   A model of interpersonal skill.

A MODEL OF INTERPERSONAL SKILL

Interpersonal skills are complex and are made up of different elements. They operate within personal, social, environmental and cultural contexts. Figure 1.2 illustrates a simple model.

More detailed models, incorporating the same assumptions, can be found in Kagan (1985) and Kagan, Evans and Kay (1986).

In the book we cover the fundamental processes of interpersonal skill, including self-awareness, social behaviour (language and non-verbal behaviour), social perception and social problem solving. We go on to consider the more complex skills of rapport, facilitation, influence and assertion, all of which combine these elements. We proceed to discuss the more complex skills still of counselling, handling conflict aggression and violence, breaking bad news and managing change. The managerial interpersonal skills of handling pressure, supervision, appraisal and performance review follow. Finally, constraints on the effective use of interpersonal skills are discussed. Each chapter is fully referenced to both social psychological and nursing literature and some ideas for further skill development are given.

CHAPTER 2

Self and self-awareness

Self-awareness is a vital part of professional interpersonal skills (French, 1983; Johnson, 1986; Kagan, 1985). Our knowledge of 'self' acts as a guide, in helping us choose our actions, the situations we meet, and the relationships we enter (Snyder, 1987). Our past experiences, current circumstances and future hopes and expectations all contribute to our feelings, attitudes, values and beliefs. These in turn affect what we do, what we notice about and how we interpret other people's behaviour. As Burnard (1989) says, in the context of counselling relationships, self-awareness allows us to:

- discriminate between our own problems and those of a 'client';
- draw boundaries between ourselves and 'clients';
- prevent emotional and physical exhaustion, or burnout;
- bring clarity and precision to the relationship by learning to choose and reflect on our responses;
- develop enhanced sensitivity to the other person's needs.

Understanding our reactions to what other people say and do, and, indeed what we ourselves say and do, and why, is the key to effective interpersonal skills (Kagan, 1981), particularly those underpinning helping relationships.

Consider, for example, the young mother who wants to talk about how to ensure her toddler eats a balanced diet. The Health Visitor will be of little help if she cannot get the pain of her sister's distress when she was a teenager, and had anorexia, out of her mind; or if she worries that she is herself becoming obsessive about food; or if her son has recently developed diabetes and she is preoccupied about whether or not he will be able to control his diet; or if she thinks the mother feeds the baby on inappropriate food (i.e. not the food that she herself would choose).

Self-awareness is a process that takes place over time, and most of us need some kind of support and help in developing it. Those professions that rely on the effective use of interpersonal skill, or that are emotionally demanding, should offer opportunities for staff to enhance their self-awareness as one aspect of enhancing their professional interpersonal skills. Supervision, mentoring and appraisal are all formal systems wherein we can enhance our self-awareness (Butterworth and Faugier, 1992; Hawkins and Shohet, 1989); informal methods may include discussion, seeking feedback from others, introspection, audio- or videotape recording of professional practice and structured exercises (Kagan, Evans and Kay, 1986; Johnson, 1986).

There are a number of different aspects of the self-system that can be brought into conscious awareness. These relate to any or all of the following:

- **Personal identity**, i.e., Who am I? How did I get to be who I am? Where do I fit in the social world?;
- **Internal events**, i.e., physiological sensations, feelings, emotions, thoughts, values, attitudes, beliefs, knowledge, understanding;
- **External events**, i.e., behaviour, speech, roles (jobs, membership of clubs, relationships, etc.);
- **Sense of self as 'agent'**, i.e., the extent to which we believe we can control events or things that happen to us.

PERSONAL IDENTITY

There are a number of different perspectives on the nature of personal identity. Psychodynamic perspectives would suggest that the 'self' is the essence of the adult person – even personality – and that identity is formed as a result of significant events that have occurred during our childhood and adolescence (Erickson, 1950; Rogers, 1961). An alternative, but not incompatible, view is that offered by symbolic interactionism. From this perspective, our identities are formed through interaction with others: the ways other people act towards us give us information about the kinds of people we are (Cooley, 1902; Mead, 1934). The first approach suggests that our sense of identity in adulthood is quite stable, and the second suggests that identity is constantly changing. Snyder (1987), however, points to differences among us in the stability of our self-systems. He distinguishes between those of us who are characterized by a 'pragmatic' self – one which adjusts to different situations – and those of us characterized by a 'principled' self that varies little in different situations.

Other theorists, however, offer frameworks for understanding identity that include both stability and change (Harré, 1984). Membership of different groups also contributes to our sense of identity (Tajfel, 1982a) and, as group membership changes, so does identity. Of course, to an extent, we choose which groups to belong to, so we determine our own identity (see 'self-as-agent' below).

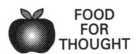

FOOD FOR THOUGHT

Is there a difference between 'self' and 'personality'? If so, what is it?

Would your answers to the question 'who am I?' be the same this year as last year? Will they be the same in five years' time? What differences might there be?

Do you let other people know your 'self' or 'personality'? How?

How consistent are you in different situations? Why is this, do you think?

'Role' and 'group' powerfully influence our sense of self. Sometimes role(s) and group(s) coincide, and then their influence is even greater.

Consider, for instance being a student nurse (role), living in a house with other student nurses (group), working with student nurses (role), being friends with student nurses (role), going on holiday with these friends (group) etc. In these circumstances, '(student) nurse' will become an important feature of one's identity. Indeed, the wearing of uniforms increases the visibility of the group, and encourages people to relate in terms of group- and role-membership, rather than as individual people. This may be one reason why, even when we wear name badges, patients still call us 'Nurse'. They are talking to us in terms of our role, and as members of the group 'nurses', from their role and membership of the group of 'patients'. If the same patients call all workers on the ward 'Nurse', they are distinguishing between themselves as belonging in the group of 'not nurse' and everyone else as belonging in the group 'nurse'.

Many of the trappings of hospitals, the illnesses that people may have, as well as nursing procedures, help remove people's sense of identity and individuality. This process of de-individuation (Diener, 1980) can lead to distorted behaviour. In the absence of self-awareness, personal identity cannot be preserved and de-individuation avoided.

Unless we have learnt to become self-aware, thinking about ourselves can lead to unpleasant feelings of self-consciousness (Buss, 1980), as the first things we notice are those things we do not like about ourselves. We have to practise self-awareness to be able to identify our strengths and positive qualities.

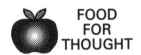

FOOD
FOR
THOUGHT

How easy do you find it to think of positive things about yourself? Why is this?

Would your parents or good friends find it easier to identify good things about you? Why?

How many of your positive qualities have you determined for yourself? How did you do this?

What effect has being a nurse had on your positive qualities?

How important have family, friends, and colleagues been in helping you see your good points?

INTERNAL EVENTS

We learn to recognize and label internal bodily states through the guesses that adults make throughout our childhood. There is, therefore, wide variation in our capacity to recognize and label these internal states accurately. We all find it difficult at times to label our bodily sensations, although we can learn to do so. This is the essence of bio-feedback techniques, whereby we learn to pick up different physiological changes. It is also the essential ingredient of many relaxation and stress reduction techniques (Murphy, 1983). If we feel nauseous following a bout of sickness and diarrhoea: is it the sickness or is it hunger that we are feeling?

The context in which we experience the sensations partly determines the label we give to them. The case is similar for the labelling of emotional states (Strongman, 1979). In general, the physiological changes underlying different emotional states are the same, but our thoughts, the context and the explanations we give for feeling as we do all help us to find a label for our feelings (Antaki, 1981; Schachter and Singer, 1962). The way we explain our feelings, or the attributions we make for our internal states can then go on to influence how we feel, even in the absence of any direct physiological arousal (Harré, 1986; Nisbett and Schachter, 1966; Valins, 1972). It is not only positive feelings that are influenced by the context and by our cognitions. The amount of pain experienced, stress, symptoms of illness (with no organic cause), dislike of particular patients and so on can all be exacerbated or alleviated by the context, our thoughts and understanding (Gildea, 1949; Hayward, 1975; Jacobson and McGrath, 1983; Moss, 1986; Stockwell, 1972).

Consider a nurse in the Accident and Emergency department. It is 11.45 pm on a Friday night. A month ago she was badly hurt by a drunk man about this time on a Friday night. She is asked to see a man who has just come in, having been involved in a street fight. What is she feeling as she goes to him and her pulse begins to race – compassion, nervousness, fear, or anger? **Her thoughts** ('How dare drunks use up scarce NHS resources!', or 'Oh no, not again . . .' or 'Poor thing, he is probably an innocent victim') may result in anger, fear or compassion respectively. When she goes to his cubicle, and finds him shouting loudly, she may be afraid because of **his behaviour**. However, when she discovers that he is profoundly deaf and has learning disabilities, the anger may go, as **the context** has now given her another way of explaining his behaviour that is not to do with him being physically threatening. So, in the course of a very short time, she may have been feeling a number of different emotions, although her level of physiological arousal may have remained about the same.

Sometimes we may feel sensations that are difficult to understand; at other times we may even be unaware of the sensations themselves. Many training programmes designed to help people reduce their anxiety or stress levels include parts that help them notice when they are becoming anxious or stressed (Looker and Gregson, 1989; Owens and Ashcroft, 1985; Pope, 1986; Trower, Bryant and Argyle, 1978). Once the signs can be noticed, they can be understood better and ways of coping may be found.

Attitudes

Attitudes are internal events that are, too, difficult to identify at times. Attitudes consist of positive or negative feelings or thoughts about an object, person or issue (Petty and Cacioppo, 1981; Fishbein and Ajzen, 1975). So, statements such as 'I like Sister Brown', 'I think disposable bedpans are a good thing', 'I hate being on nights and think there should always be a qualified member of staff on every ward', are all expressions of attitudes. Attitudes are, however, hypothetical constructs, in that they cannot be seen, and we simply infer from them what we think, feel and do, although there have been many attempts to measure them (Stahlberg and Frey, 1988). The relationship between attitudes and behaviour is an interesting one. What does it mean, for instance when the nurse who says she likes Sister Brown runs and hides whenever she approaches; or when the nurse who hails the advent of disposable bedpans always uses metal ones; or when the student nurse who professes to dislike nights always volunteers for extra night duty? A great deal of research has been carried out, demonstrating to greater or lesser extents the consistencies between attitudes, and between attitudes and behaviour. Other work has recommended the abandonment of the search for consistency: instead, the extent of inconsistency, and the circumstances giving rise to inconsistencies, are better subjects for scrutiny (Antaki, 1988; Billig *et al.*, 1988). Nevertheless, we may well ask what social meanings attitudes have if particular behaviours are not linked to them.

Just as we can have attitudes towards other people (we shall be considering strong attitudes towards others, or prejudices, as well as attempts to change them, in Chapter 5), so we have attitudes towards ourselves. If we have strong positive attitudes towards ourselves (that is, we think highly of and like ourselves), we are said to have **high self-esteem**: if we have strong negative attitudes towards ourselves (that is, we think badly of and dislike ourselves), we are said to have **low self-esteem** (Argyle, 1983). Most people are happier and more confident in their daily lives if they have high self-esteem (Rowe, 1983). We shall see later that level of self-esteem is affected by our sense of self as 'agent'.

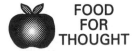

FOOD FOR THOUGHT

What characteristics do you share with people you admire and those you do not admire?

> Why is it that you admire (or not) the things you do in other people?
>
> How do you think your best friend might see you in terms of these characteristics?
>
> What makes you feel good about yourself? Does anyone else know this about you? Why/why not?
>
> What stops you being more like your idea of an 'ideal' person?

One of the most important ways we form views of ourselves is by comparing ourselves with others (Festinger, 1954). How similar to people we like are we? How similar to people we dislike are we? Sometimes we get an idea of someone, or a group of people we aspire to be like; we then try to adopt the characteristics or behaviours that would make us more like this 'reference group' (Turner and Giles, 1981). So, the child who wants to be a nurse will use 'nurses' as her/his reference group to give her/him some idea of how to act, and so on. Similarly, the nurse who had really wanted to be a doctor may try to act like one. (It is interesting to consider why some nurses, psychologists and so on, who have a PhD, call themselves 'Doctor' when they work in hospital settings. There is no reason why they should not – but what does doing so reveal about their concept of 'self'?)

Comparisons with others, then, is vital for our sense of identity and self-esteem (Rijsman, 1983). Equally important are our values and beliefs.

Values and beliefs

In nursing the values and beliefs we hold will affect our reactions to different situations, as well as guide our behaviour in general. Indeed, our values and beliefs may be what took us into nursing in the first place. Values are implicit or explicit views about what we consider to be ideal, or about desirable ways of achieving these ideals. We each hold a small number of values, making up a values set. By and large these values are consistent: they are central to our personal being and provide us with a sense of moral direction (Maslow, 1971; Rogers, 1980). Values may also contribute to our cultural or subcultural ident-ities. As George and Wilding (1985) point out, people may not always behave according to their value sets, but at times they are prepared to die for them. Awareness of our values helps us see what is and is not acceptable to us in the context of our work (Beardshaw, 1981). There is a current interest in so-called 'whistle-blowers' working in the health service. 'Whistle-blowing' occurs when people consider their values to have been compromised to such an extent that their jobs are no longer more important than speaking out.

At a personal level, many values are underpinned by 'social needs', such as a need to be liked, a need to be needed and a need for power (Maslow, 1970). When these values are challenged, we may become, for example, defensive, aggressive, despondent or insensitive.

Consider the friendly nurse who 'needs to be liked', but whose patients seem ungrateful and dismissive; she may feel a sense of rejection or frustration. The nurse who 'needs to achieve' may act in ways to get himself noticed, rather than in the best interests of patients. The nurse who has a 'need for power' may change when prospects for promotion appear. He may forgo his erstwhile values of 'equality' and 'honesty', and replace them with values of 'self-interest' and 'expediency'. He may insist on doing only those tasks that will get him noticed: he may put on a different face when senior staff are around and may cut off long-standing friendships if they might detract from his possibility of promotion. The community nurse who has a 'need to be needed' may be blinkered to the fact that her patient no longer benefits from nursing care, and still carry on visiting.

Values, then bring consistency to our behaviour, and give us a sense of personal and cultural identity. They are resistant to change, but whenever changes do occur, they will lead to widespread change in our behaviour.

Beliefs are opinion linked to values, from which attitudes will stem. They, too, are thought to be highly resistant to change. A change in our fundamental beliefs is usually the result of some experience that has a profound effect on us and will inevitably change many of the ways we behave. Changes in other beliefs may occur more easily, and have little effect. Different types of belief are summarized in Table 2.1.

Attitudes, values and beliefs about health and illness, as well as about suitable treatments, will influence the interpersonal skills of nurses, patients, employers and other health workers (Marteau, 1989). Similarities in attitudes, values or beliefs may make interpersonal situations go smoothly; differences in attitudes, values or beliefs may disrupt, or even destroy, interpersonal relationships.

Table 2.1 Types of belief and consequences of change (from Kagan, Evans and Kay, 1986, after Rokeach, 1968)

Type of belief	Source of belief	Example	Change
Shared privitive beliefs	Widely held in a particular culture	I believe in the sanctity of life	Difficult – leading to trauma
Unshared primitive beliefs	Self-identity and personal experience	I believe men should have equal responsibility for child care	Difficult – leading to widespread changes
Authority beliefs	Derived from (perceived) legitimate authority (e.g. the hospital authorities)	I believe staffing levels in the NHS should be maintained (after all it's district policy)	Can change with perceived legitimacy of the authority or with changing experiences
Derived beliefs	Derived from authorities with which individual identifies (e.g. another valued person)	I believe in giving patients the option to have electro-convulsive shock treatment (that's what my tutor believes)	Can change with changing experiences, and often through communication
Inconsequential beliefs	Past experience, prejudices, etc.	I believe this ward always gets the post last	Easily changed – pervasive effects

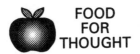

**FOOD
FOR
THOUGHT**

Can you identify three of your fundamental beliefs and values about nursing: where do they each come from?

What would it take to change any of these beliefs or values?

Do values and beliefs vary with culture, age, or sex? In what ways?

Are some people's belief systems more rigid than others? Are these people more predictable than others?

Are some people's value sets less consistent than others? Does this have any impact on their behaviour?

Is there anything about nurse training that attempts to change beliefs about nursing? How successful is it?

EXTERNAL EVENTS

On the whole, we are aware of how we talk and behave, which clubs we belong to and why. What we may not be aware of is the information these external events give other people about our own identity. It is sometimes said that we each have 'public' and 'private' selves (Buss, 1980). We take care to present our 'public' selves in ways that give different information to different groups of people (Goffman, 1959). The book we choose to read on the train, the clothes we choose to wear to a party or job interview, the way we greet the Unit General Manager, will all reveal different aspects of our 'self' to the different audiences. The more involved with a role we are (with all the attendant 'props', like uniforms, equipment, etc.), or the more restricted we are by our place in a particular social system, or the more clear the rules guiding our behaviour are, the less personal information we reveal (Goffman 1967, 1971; Herzlich, 1974; Parsons, 1951; Totman, 1979). Thus it may be hard to get to know much about the way individual patients really think and feel if they are fully immersed in a 'sick role' (Mayou, 1984; Mechanic, 1986). An optimistic view of both primary nursing (Wright, 1990) and the nursing process is that they both enable role barriers to be broken down, so that people meet as **people**, and not as 'nurses', 'patients, and so on.

Self-presentation

Our attempts to present our 'selves' in different ways have been likened to drama (Goffman, 1967; Harré, 1993). It is as if we are all actors on a stage, playing different roles at all times, however informally, to different audiences. The roles we take and our interpretation of them depend on the situation and the scripts we are expected (by our other actors and by our audience) to follow. Extending our analogy with the theatre, there are 'on-stage' and 'backstage' areas. We perform publicly, in order to give particular impressions to our audience, when we are on-stage, but drop our 'mask' when we return to the more private backstage.

Consider the community nurse who behaves with bristling efficiency on a home visit, in front of her 'audience' of patient and family, and who becomes deflated and slow with exhaustion when she believes herself to be alone in her car, only to become dynamic when visiting her next family. She is treating the home situations as 'on-stage' and her car as 'backstage'. Should she see someone she knows, while in her car, she will quickly try to gain an on-stage appearance.

The argument, then, is that we try to present different facets of 'self' in different lights on different occasions. Our choice of how we do this depends largely on how we perceive ourselves, that is, the kind of person we think we are and would like others to think we are. It does not always happen like this: sometimes we try to hide the kind of person we think we are by presenting ourselves in particular ways. Even if we present ourselves in ways that are 'not really us', other people's reactions may mean that is how we become after all. If we pick up a discrepancy between how we think of ourselves and how others seem to be expecting us to be, or even between our own expectations of ourselves and our actual selves, we may become depressed (Kovacs and Beck, 1978).

It can sometimes be surprising to find out what kind of a person other people think we are. Generally, we pick up cues about the impressions we make on others from the ways they behave towards us – although, of course, we may be wrong.

Subjective and objective self-awareness

Goffman writes from a symbolic interactionist perspective (Cuff, Sharrock and Francis, 1992). Symbolic interactionism describes a num-

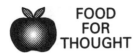

**FOOD
FOR
THOUGHT**

Try to imagine what a) someone you know quite well, but do not like, b) someone of the opposite sex, c) someone a lot older or younger than you thinks you are like. How do you know what they think?

Is this what you would like them to think of you? If not, what might you do to alter their perceptions?

What kinds of characteristics have you thought about? Why these ones?

Do you think a good friend would use the same characteristics in describing the kind of person you are? Why/why not?

How do you form impressions of others? How easily changed are your judgements?

What roles do values, attitudes and beliefs play in making judgements about others?

ber of different approaches that all share an interest in the ways that people actively negotiate actions, through the use of symbols, in particular language. Our sense of self is a product of interaction with others, and at the same time determines this interaction. Thus social experience is fundamental to our sense of self and *vice versa*. Mead (1934), drawing on earlier philosophical work, suggests that the 'self' is both object (the **me** – derived from other people's attitudes and behaviour), and subject (the **I** – the individual's inner response to other people's attitudes). By taking on those attitudes of others towards us (the **me**), the **I** reacts. It is suggested that this capacity of ours to be reflexive, i.e., able to reflect upon aspects of ourselves, is one of the things that makes us able to understand ourselves and each other.

To say that we are able to think carefully about the ways we present ourselves to others is not to imply that we are continually self-aware. Certainly, when we are deciding what to wear one day, or are thinking about how happy or upset we might be, we are in a state of self-awareness. We are **subjectively self-aware**, in so far as we are aware of our internal thoughts or feelings. Every now and then, though, something happens to make us aware of ourselves as other people see us. We are then **objectively self-aware** (Duval and Wicklund, 1972).

Often, as a result of becoming objectively self-aware, we notice our own deficiencies, and this may lead to us doing something differently ('I must get a haircut/watch my accent/give the injection more slowly,

Consider the ways we might become objectively self-aware. We might catch sight of ourselves in the back of a metal bedpan as we are emptying it; we may see a photograph of ourselves taken by the local reporter doing an article about our health centre; or we may hear a tape-recording of ourselves after putting a report for a case conference on to a Dictaphone. In all these examples, we might ask ourselves 'Is that how I appear to other people?'. Other ways of becoming objectively self-aware are when we are, or think we are, being watched, examined or judged in some way. A mother wanting us remove her son's stitches is potentially judging us. If we are conducting an interview in a side room which has a video recorder and camera stored in it, there is the potential for being videoed, and found wanting by a (potential) audience. We may anticipate what someone else would think of us if they saw us ('What would Sister think of the way I am giving this injection?').

etc.'). We do differ, though, in the extent to which we are aware of either internal of external events. Some people are painfully aware of themselves and their shortcomings and are likely to be self-conscious as a result; others are impervious to even their largest 'imperfections', and certainly to others' reactions to them and they may well be arrogant or overly self-confident (Buss, 1980). Happily, most of us fall somewhere between realistic self-appraisal and the motivation to change some things about our 'selves'.

As nurses, positive feedback from people that coincides with how we feel about ourselves will make us feel good and enjoy our work. Negative feedback from others that contradicts how we see ourselves will make us miserable and dissatisfied with work. Ironically, the public's expectations of nurses frequently contradicts our own perceptions of ourselves and our jobs; this becomes more apparent to students as they progress although training and often contributes to increasing dissatisfaction with the job (Llewelyn, 1984, 1989). Similarly, the mismatch between patients' expectations of nurses in, say, intensive therapy units (to make comfortable and to reassure), with the nurses' tasks of administering some painful treatment (such as coughing and aspiration after thoracic surgery) may lead to patient dissatisfaction.

SENSE OF SELF AS 'AGENT'

We have seen, above, that our feelings about ourselves are determined, in part, by the ways in which other people react towards us. Furthermore, we try to control the impression they get of us by presenting ourselves in particular ways. In order to have self-confidence and to act effectively, we must believe that we can control how others see us. In addition, we must believe that we can exert some control over our environments (Steiner, 1981) and our own efficacy (Bandura, 1978). In other words, we have to believe in ourselves as 'agents', and not as objects to be controlled by others (Harré, 1993, 1984), although this is not necessarily so in all cultures (Marsella, DeVos and Hsu, 1985). If we experience little or no control over our environments, our health and morale may decline, leading to illness, depression and even, it has been suggested, death. It is suggested that, faced with no control over events, we learn to be helpless (Brown and Harris, 1978; Glass and Singer, 1972; Peterson and Seligman, 1984; Rowe, 1983). However, it is the belief that we have control, rather than the control itself, that is thought to lead to psychological and physical wellbeing, self-confidence and high self-esteem. As Niven (1989) points out, when the perception of the control is lost, stress and anxiety often follow.

Perceived lack of control

Perceived lack of control, leading to the kinds of passivity mentioned above, often characterizes people who are ill and who think there is nothing they can do about it. A different effect is found if we want to control our health, or think we should control it. We may fight the apparent lack of control we find when we do not get better, or when health workers try to make us submit to a particular treatment, and display what is known as 'reactance' (Worchel and Brehm, 1971). Reactance can occur whenever we find ourselves unable to control events that we expect to be able to, or when we think we are being denied freedom of choice.

Consider the obese patient who has been put on a diet prior to a hip replacement. Even though he has lost a lot of weight he goes on an eating binge. His freedom of choice has been restricted (albeit for his own good), and he displays reactance. The binge is an attempt to regain control. Consider too, the mother of a young man who has developed symptoms of schizophrenia. As the years go by, nothing the health service can offer seems to make any difference. The mother does not give up and travels abroad in search of promised 'cures'. She thinks she should be able to find something that will help him, and in the face of being unable to, tries all the harder. This is not a denial of her son's difficulties – as might be suggested – but rather reactance.

Perceived lack of control can lead to stress (Glass and Singer, 1972; Rowe, 1983). The different reactions we have to lack of control is partly due to our different reactions to stress. Working in a context where we have little autonomy is likely to be stressful, and we will experience a weak sense of 'self as agent'. Hospitals are good at denying patients and staff alike choices over all manner of things to do with their daily lives, and this contributes to both apathy and aggression.

Consider a long-stay ward: patients cannot choose how to place the furniture; (sometimes) what they have on the tops of their lockers; whether to get up or to stay in bed; (sometimes) what they have to eat (even if there is ostensibly a choice of menu, their 'order' does not always arrive); when to have a bath, what to wear and so on. Staff may not be able to choose when to talk to whom (or when not to); when to have a cup of tea; what to do; what to wear and so on. Consequently they may feel at the end of the day that they have been shoved about by other people, and are 'nobodies'.

Not only is it important, then, to retain a sense of 'self as agent' ourselves, but also to give other people opportunities to retain their sense of 'self as agent'.

The processes involved in the different reactions to perceived lack of control are shown in Figure 2.1.

The importance of self as 'agent' has been studied in a culture where an individual's freedom of choice and expression is highly valued. In cultures where co-operation and collective or social identity has pre-

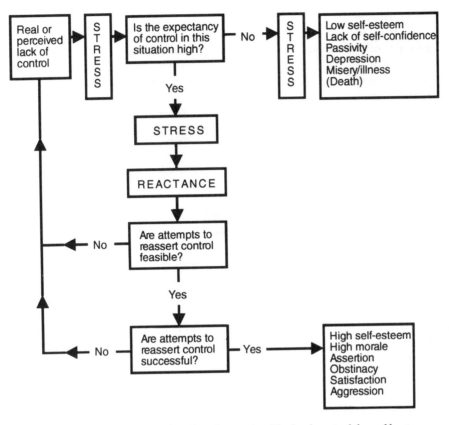

Figure 2.1 Consequences of real and perceived lack of control for self-esteem: sense of self as 'agent' (from Kagan, Evans and Kay, 1986).

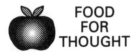 **FOOD FOR THOUGHT**

Think of a recent time when your lack of control led to a) apathy and b) reactance.

What attempts did you make to regain control?

How did you feel?

Would your reactions have been the same if the other main people involved had been of the opposite sex/20 years older/from a different culture? Why/why not?

How much of your reaction was due to you, and how much to the situation?

cedence over individual identity, people may not respond to loss of agency in the same ways. Self as 'agent' may feature more or less prominently in various cultures and/or subcultures. Certainly, if we take seriously the idea that self is a social product, we would expect women, people with disabilities, people from different communities or nations, blacks, people with different sexual orientations, and so on, to respond to greater lack of agency in different ways (Adams, 1989; Campling, 1981; Fanon, 1986; Hogg and Abrams, 1988; Marsella, DeVos and Hsu, 1985; Morris, 1991).

Consider the possibility that people who are used to having a lot of control or social power might be the ones to react most strongly to lack of control. If this is so, it might be that teachers, company directors, politicians and doctors, for example, make particularly 'bad' patients. Furthermore, they should be at their worst when they are feeling relatively well, but restrictions are imposed upon them, such as enforced immobility following orthopaedic surgery.

THE PROCESS OF BECOMING SELF-AWARE

We said earlier that self-awareness was not achieved once and for all, but rather that it was a continuing process. It has been argued that one of the main purposes of life is to strive for a state of self-actualization (Rogers, 1961, 1980), and self-awareness is one of the means of achieving this. We become healthier and happier if we can be aware of ourselves and be open and honest in our transactions with other people (Johnson, 1986). Only when we are able to do this, and to integrate all our experiences – past, present and future – into our self-system, will we be able to help others effectively. The idea is not that increased self-awareness will lead us to become paragons of virtue, or even boringly self-occupied, as is often feared. Instead, self-awareness should enable us to see when our own concerns obstruct our abilities to listen and respond to other people effectively. Without self-awareness, our own insecurities, fears, preferences, preoccupations and so on can lead us to block what we, or others, say or do, as well as to misinterpret what we see or hear. We can only remove the obstructions when we are able to recognize them in the first place. As we have seen, self-awareness comes about largely through our relations with

	Known to self	Unknown to self
Known to others	**a Public self** What I know and I present to others so that they know it too	**b Blind self** Those aspects of me that I am unaware of but that others see and judge me by
Unknown to others	**c Private self** What I know but I do not want other people to know or to discover	**d Unknown self** What I do not know, or do not (want to) recognize, and that others are not aware of

The process of self-awareness means that those aspects known to 'self' are increased. Sometimes the 'private' area will also be decreased, for example:

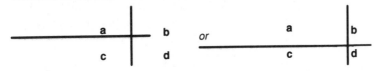

Figure 2.2 The process of self-awareness through self-knowledge and feedback from other people: the Johari window (from Kagan, Evans and Kay, 1986).

other people: while this is a continual and natural process, we can speed it up by concentrating on our learning from spoken and unspoken messages, as well as opening ourselves to share our self-knowledge with others.

Joe Luft and Harry Ingham summarize the process of becoming self-aware through feedback from others and self-disclosure in what has become known as the Johari Window (from Joe and Harry!) (Luft, 1969; Pfeiffer and Jones, 1974). Figure 2.2 shows the way the Johari window can contribute to self-awareness.

We will never achieve total self-awareness (how would we know we had achieved it, anyway?), but can work at making constructive use of our experiences throughout life, in order to enhance our personal relationships and make more effective use of our professional inter-personal skills.

SUMMARY

This chapter has been concerned with the central place of self and self-awareness in interpersonal skill. Specifically, the following issues were raised:

- Self-awareness is a key component of interpersonal skill.
- Self-awareness takes place over time.

- Personal identity, internal and external events and the sense of self as 'agent' contribute to self-awareness.
- Personal identity develops throughout life, is moulded by our understanding of how other people see us and changes with group membership.
- If personal identity is undermined we may experience de-individuation.
- Contexts and experience help us recognize and label internal states.
- Attitudes, values and beliefs are important internal events which contribute to our sense of self.
- Values affect our experiences of many work practices, and may be linked to social needs.
- Values and fundamental beliefs are highly resistant to change, whereas other beliefs and attitudes may be changed more easily.
- We each have public and private selves.
- Public selves are presented in different ways to different groups of people and in different situations.
- Self-presentation varies according to the situation and the role we are playing.
- Symbolic interactionism stresses the meanings we convey about ourselves in different situations, and that others convey to us about ourselves.
- A distinction can be drawn between self-as-subject (**I**) and self-as-object (**Me**).
- We are subjectively self-aware if we are aware of internal events, and objectively self-aware if we are aware of how others see us.
- Real or perceived control over events leads to a sense of 'agency'.
- Without a sense of 'agency' we may feel helpless, stressed and anxious.
- If control is taken away from us, we may try to regain it by resisting attempts to get us to do things (i.e., we may display reactance).
- Self-awareness, openness and honesty in interpersonal encounters can make us feel more fulfilled.
- Self-awareness can lead to greater interpersonal effectiveness.

SELF-DEVELOPMENT EXERCISES

1. Give 20 answers to the question 'Who am I?' Look at your lists and put 'R' by answers that are roles (for example, 'I am a nurse/a sister/a church warden'); put 'D' by any that are descriptions (for example, 'I am tall/happy/female'); put 'G' by any that denote membership of a group (for example, 'I am a member of a primary health care team/a student/a care manager'). Consider the overlap

between and relative importance of descriptions, roles and group membership for personal and social identity.

2. Ask three friends how they think children learn to identify emotions. How might you discover whether or not they are right?
3. Interview a colleague about a time s/he found it difficult to cope. Try to discover the extent to which s/he thought about the ability of other people to cope in similar circumstances. What was the effect of knowing how other people managed on her/his self-confidence?
4. List your core attitudes, values and beliefs. Which of your attitudes and values come from influences in your childhood and which come from your adult life experiences?
5. Discuss with colleagues your 'bottom line' in terms of those things you are not willing to compromise on in your nursing practice. How does compromise affect morale?
6. Take any social situation you have been in recently. Can you describe it as if it were a theatrical performance? Identify the actors, audience, roles, scripts, props, on-stage and backstage regions. How useful is a dramaturgical approach to the analysis of self-awareness?
7. How do you present yourself in different social situations? Consider both your appearance and your behaviour. How deliberate is your self-presentation?
8. Find a way of being part of a large crowd (in, for example, a theatre, city centre before Christmas). How does it feel? Is it easier or more difficult to be uninhibited if you are with people you know? How do you retain a sense of your own individuality in the crowd?

CHAPTER 3

Social behaviour

If we are to use interpersonal skills we must engage in social behaviour. It can be useful to consider both verbal and non-verbal aspects of social behaviour (see Figure 1.2), although it is essential to remember that in most cases the two 'systems' are interrelated in complex ways. At times, though, one system may be dominant. In noisy environments, or when relating to people who have lost their hearing, permanently or temporarily, the non-verbal channel assumes dominance: in those situations where vision is attenuated, or permanently lost, the verbal channel assumes dominance. Sometimes, too, when ambiguous messages are given out (that is the person says something, but her/his body 'says' the opposite), one or other channel will be noticed more, depending on the situation. The distinction between verbal and non-verbal channels can also be made in relation to both the observation and interpretation of other people's behaviour.

NON-VERBAL BEHAVIOUR

We use the term 'non-verbal behaviour' here to refer to anything about social performance that is not speech, or the actual words that are spoken. We have said above that under normal circumstances non-verbal communication is not a separate communication system. Rather, it relates to speech in several different ways: non-verbal messages may enhance the meaning of what is said, synchronize conversation, obtain feedback on what is being said, signal interest and attentiveness, replace (as in sign language), or contradict the verbal messages (Argyle, 1983). It is usually the non-verbal cues that we notice first on meeting people. On the basis of this information we form impressions about the other person's values and attitudes, personality, interests, and so on; as Strongman (1979, p. 213) says 'Any judgements that we make about people are all made as inferences from what they look like and what they do'. In fact we make judgements very quickly about the kind of person we think she or he is. (We shall see later that these judgements are as much about our expectations and interpretations and may or may not be correct, but we make then nevertheless!) At the same time, by the ways we present ourselves, we are giving a lot of information to others that may lead them to make judgements about our own values and attitudes and the kinds of people we are (Goffman, 1959).

The different categories of non-verbal behaviour are listed below.

A taxonomy of non-verbal behaviour

Facial expression
Eyebrows
Nose
Cheeks
Forehead
Mouth
Eye movements
Eye region
Mouth region
Tongue

Proximity and touch
Patterns of bodily accessibility
Personal distance
Ritual/task-related physical contact
Touching self (scratching, rubbing, twiddling hair/rings, etc.)

Posture, orientation and gait
Position of limbs/head
Position of body
Regularity of movements
Speed/regularity of walking

Artefacts
Appearance: dress, cosmetics, hair, accessories (e.g., bags, spectacles, jewellery), cleanliness, smell
Emblems: badges, uniforms, possessions (make of car, newspaper, etc.)

Gesture
Hand
Head – shake, nod, toss
Facial
Arm
Body
Leg/foot
Vocal

Eye gaze
Eye contact
Direction of gaze
Staring
Duration of gaze
Avoidance
Blinking

Vocal
Tone and pitch
Clarity
Pauses
Dysfluencies
Volume
Amount
Hesitation
Sighs
Speed
Silence
Verbal cliches
Laughs

Note: Combinations of non-verbal behaviours mean different things, and **movement** changes the meaning

Generally, we assume that all behaviour means something, and react accordingly. We usually base our decisions about meaning on what we would expect the behaviour to mean, given the particular cultural and situational context in which it occurred (Forgas, 1985b).

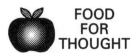

FOOD FOR THOUGHT

Can you note down non-verbal behaviours when two people are talking? What difficulties does this raise?

Are some non-verbal behaviours easier to identify than others? Why?

How closely linked are non-verbal behaviours to the topics of conversation?

What non-verbal behaviours do you think you display?

Do people of different ages use different non-verbal behaviours? In what ways?

How do the non-verbal behaviours of women and men differ?

Non-verbal habits

As we saw in Chapter 1, one assumption behind viewing interpersonal behaviour as a skill is that it is learnt. Thus we have learnt to behave in particular ways non-verbally (and verbally), usually responding differently in different situations Bandura (1977). What we display at any particular point in time, however, may be a habit, rather than a meaningful communication. The trouble is, though, other people may interpret our habits in various ways.

Consider, for example, Ann, who is 13 and is admitted to a paediatric ward because she has lost two-thirds of her body weight. She smiles and giggles a lot when discussing her condition. The nurses tell her consultant she thinks the whole business is very funny and does not recognize the seriousness of the problem. The care team agree there is no point trying to agree a strategy for weight gain with Ann and that instead they should work on helping her gain insight into her problem. What they do not know, and have made no attempt to find out, is that Ann giggles and laughs at everything in all situations. This is a habit she has developed and it does not mean anything.

As a result of their interpretations of the meaning of Ann's behaviour the care team have proposed one course of action when another may have been more useful. If Ann had said to herself 'I must stop giggling and smiling when talking to the nurses', she might well have found it more difficult to have a proper conversation. Her words might have become muddled, she might have gone 'blank' or some other non-verbal behaviours might have appeared or changed.

Habits are difficult to change. Once we try to change any part of our interpersonal behaviour, the system as a whole may be upset.

Still, it is worth trying to change those habits of ours that we know detract from effective use of interpersonal skills, but we should bear in mind (and be prepared to deal with) the other (unintended) changes that may occur.

The regulation of encounters

Non-verbal behaviours help regulate encounters. Argyle (1983) suggests they do this in a number of ways; by:

- controlling synchronization (that is, ensuing a smooth pattern of turn-taking in conversation, especially via shifts of gaze, head nods and grunts);
- obtaining feedback (that is gaining information on how others respond – whether they understand, are interested or bored, agree or disagree and so on. Head nods and changes in facial expression or body orientation give this information);
- signalling attentiveness (that is, giving intermittent messages that others are being attended to via body orientation, head nods, intermittent eye contact, congruent posture and minimal vocalizations).

When some of these channels of non-verbal communication are closed (for example, when people talk on the telephone) the interactions will often go less smoothly. People will interrupt each other more and it may be difficult to end the conversation. The person who has more non-verbal information will usually dominate the conversation.

The use of speech is inextricably linked to certain aspects of non-verbal behaviour, particularly those in the 'paralinguistic' category.

Consider, for example, the many situations in which nurses have more non-verbal information than patients do. Talking from the end of the bed to patients who are lying down, talking to people with visual or hearing impairments, talking to people who are temporarily handicapped by a dressing or medical procedure depriving them of sight hearing or touch are all such situations. It would be very easy for nurses to dominate the conversation either by talking more or by asking more questions. They are very likely, too, to have more sustained eye contact, possibly making patients feel uncomfortable. It is a real challenge for nurses to find ways of putting such patients (or relatives) at their ease and helping them be more equal in the conversation.

SPEECH

We can consider speech at a range of different levels, from sounds, syllables, words, phases, sentences, to sequences, and so on (Gahagan, 1984). For our purposes here, we will examine the social use of language, and so consider it at the level of meaning, which is inextricably linked to the influence of social variables (Forgas, 1985a). As with non-verbal behaviour, there may well be a mismatch between what the speaker intended and what the listener thought s/he meant. Most things we say have both **latent** (hidden) and **manifest** (obvious) meanings.

Consider, for example: 'What was that you said'

Manifest: 'Please repeat what you said.'
Latent: 'You're so boring, I wasn't listening.'

This example shows how language can be used to convey information beyond the surface topic of conversation. In this case the latent meaning communicates interpersonal attitudes and judgements.

Interaction	Smooth		Disrupted	
Speaker intends	LATENT		LATENT	
Listener perceives		LATENT		MANIFEST
Speaker intends	MANIFEST		MANIFEST	
Listener perceives		MANIFEST		LATENT

Figure 3.1 Interaction as a function of shared meaning (from Kagan, Evans and Kay, 1986).

Cues as to which meaning is intended are given by the expression we use and other non-verbal accompaniments, such as facial expression and timing (Hargie, Saunders and Dickson, 1981). So, at times we can intend the latent meaning to be picked up, and confusion will arise if the listener responds to the manifest meaning; at other times, however, we may intend to convey the manifest meaning, but the listener interprets what we say at the latent level, once more leading to confusion. Smooth interaction requires both listener and speaker to be operating at the same level of meaning (Figure 3.1).

As we shall see later, many of the strategies of speech we use exploit the ambiguity inherent in the two levels of meaning.

Rules of conversations

A great deal of what we say (and how we interpret what others say) is in accordance with rules (Gahagan, 1984; Goffman, 1971). These rules, which may be explicit (clearly stated) or implicit (assumed), determine the level of detail that is used, the content of what is said, the order of successive bits of speech and how the elements are related to each other. There are some general rules that govern many different aspects of interaction, but there are also rules that are specific to different situations and the roles people occupy in these situations.

Gahagan (1984, p. 55), following the work of Clark and Clark (1977), suggests that:

Conversations are bounded by the following rules:
- Each participant has a chance to talk.
- Only one person speaks at a time.
- Gaps between utterances are brief.
- Order of speaking is not fixed in advance.
- The person who initiates the conversation provides the first topic.
- The elements of a conversation consist to a considerable extent in adjacency pairs, as in the following:

Request – Grant
Assertion – Acknowledgement
Offer – Acceptance/rejection
Question – Answer.

. . . Adjacency pairs ensure that speakers observe rules of relevance when they think they are having a conversation.

If any of these rules are broken, the interaction will be disrupted and confusion may arise. However, the rules are not invariant, and both partners may not be fully aware of them. Furthermore, they are often (sub)culturally specific, and may change with the situation.

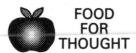

FOOD FOR THOUGHT

How easy is it to identify the rules of any conversation?
    Do you think anyone taking part in a conversation would agree what the rules are?
    Are the rules underlying some conversations easier to identify than others? Why?
    Do people of different ages and different sexes follow different conversational rules? In what ways?
    Are there missing situations that do not have rules underlying the conversations?
    How does role and setting influence conversational rules?

The breaking of the rules of conversation is often an attempt to communicate something that we find difficult to say. We need to be aware of the context in which conversations take place, in order fully to understand them.

Consider, for example, the nurse who is sensitive to the underlying message being given by the patient as s/he breaks rules of conversation:

Nurse: What did you have for dinner?
Patient: They've changed my pills. (*breaking rule of relevance*)

Nurse: Oh? Does that worry you? (*sensitive response*)
Patient: I . . . yes . . . well . . . I think it does . . . I mean. I must be getting worse, mustn't I?

This nurse, on the other hand, is insensitive:

Nurse: What did you have for dinner?
Patient: They've changed my pills. (*breaking rule of relevance*)
Nurse: You were meant to have had cod in cheese sauce. (*persisting, insensitive*)
Patient: What? . . . Oh, yes. We did.

Sometimes, just listening to, or reading what was said is misleading, as the rules of relevance may appear to have been broken, but are, in fact, unspoken, but fully understood by both participants. For example:

Patient: Can I walk to the bathroom?
Nurse: Sister will be here in a minute.

This seems to be insensitive response by the nurse, but when we know, as both patient and nurse do here, that Sister has said she wants to go with this patient when she walks to the bathroom, we see that the rules of relevance had not been broken, and that the nurse was responding appropriately. We need to be aware of the context in which conversations take place, in order fully to understand them.

Strategies of speech

Factors determining what we say and how we say it, then, depend to a large extent on the rules prescribed by the situation. The more formal the situation, the greater the constraints on who says what to whom (Goffman, 1971). Weddings, committees, and so on are examples of formal situations with predetermined rules of speech. Such regular patterns of speech that are clearly dictated by rules are known as **rituals** (Goffman, 1967; Argyle, 1983). They apply to less formal situations as well as the formal ones.

There are other social and interpersonal considerations that determine our choice of language, most of which are linked in some way to the roles we and our partner(s) fulfil (Gahagan, 1984).

The style of speech we adopt is known as the 'code', and reflects the assumptions we make about (what we take to be) the listener's state of knowledge.

Relative power and status of partners is reflected by form of address we use, and also by, for example, who is permitted to initiate conversations. So on a ward round, a 'rule' may be that the consultant can

Consider, for example, the request 'Please take this to her, over there', which assumes that the listener knows what is to be taken to whom, and the context is such that the person's whereabouts is known. Another request, however, makes no such assumption: 'Please take this haemoglobin report to Sister – she is the one in blue who is standing by the window.' The first request was made in a **restricted code** (**RC**) and the second in an **elaborated code** (**EC**). An 'outsider' would not be able to understand the RC as it assumes a great deal of prior knowledge. Talking 'shop' and using jargon are further examples of RC, and they are frequently used to convey the message 'You are not one of us'. It can be embarrassing, and even humiliating, to have to ask for elaboration of a RC, as this is tantamount to saying 'I am not familiar with you/the subject/the situation'. Consider, for example, the following:

> **Patient**: Nurse, it's time I went now. (*restricted code*)
> **Nurse**: Went where? (*request for elaboration*)
> **Patient** (to other patient): Wouldn't you know it? Just my luck – a new 'un. (*consequences for relationship*)

Explanations, or conversations with strangers, often have to be made in EC.

address a student nurse, but not *vice versa*. The 'high status' person, then, has the right to control the interaction.

We have seen that the level of precision used reflects what the speaker thinks the listener needs to know. Using RC like this can, however, lead the listener to make incorrect inferences from what is said. This can be illustrated by the following conversation.

> **Nurse 1**: Jane stayed in bed all day yesterday. (*making assumptions about listener's state of knowledge*)
> **Nurse 2**: Lazy thing! She's going the right way to get disciplined. (*making incorrect inference*)
> **Nurse 1**: But she was ill! (*retrieving the conversation by elaborating/clarifying*)

So far, we have considered language choice as the reflection of the relationship between partners. It can also create a set of relationships

(Robinson, 1972). If we deliberately talk in such a way that assumes knowledge that we know our partner does not have, we create a superior relationship. Similarly, if we elaborate our conservations, assuming our partner knows nothing, when we know s/he does have some relevant knowledge, we again create a situation of superiority. Very many strategies of speech that we use communicate relative status; even if we do not intend a 'status message' to be given, what we say may be interpreted as one.

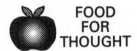

**FOOD
FOR
THOUGHT**

As you listen to conversation, can you:

- identify the goals each person has;
- identify any jargon, restricted codes, latent/manifest meanings or other strategies of speech;
- tell how the situation or the roles of the people influenced the conversation;
- identify different strategies used by people of different ages and different sexes?

The only way we really know how our partner has interpreted what we have said is by the way s/he responds and the consequences that follow for the rest of the interaction, and subsequent interactions, with the same partner. The social functions that language serves, and some of the strategies that we all use every day, are summarized in Table 3.1.

Interaction context

As we noted above, the only way we can really tell whether or not a particular strategy has fulfilled its function is by looking at the effect of using that strategy. Just to know that a joke was made is not very helpful, unless we can know that people laughed. While the intentions of a speaker are important, it is far more helpful to be able to judge the reactions of the listener accurately. Only then will we be able to make any necessary adjustments to our own behaviour – an essential component of the effective use of interpersonal skill (Argyle, 1984; French, 1983; Hargie, Saunders and Dixon, 1981; Hollin and Trower, 1986a). In taking the 'other's' reactions into account we are using what is known

Table 3.1 Social functions and strategies of speech (derived in part from Robinson, 1972 and Halliday, 1973)

Function	Focus	Strategies	Examples
Communication of relative:			
a) status	Role	'One-upmanship'	P: I broke my arm getting my parachute off.
		Name-dropping	N: When I last spoke to Professor Brown . . .
		Distraction	N: Sorry. . . . You were saying?
b) interest	Interpersonal attitudes	Formality of address	N: Good afternoon, Mrs Robinson v. Hiya, pet!
			P: Hello, Doctor!
			Chaplain: Let us pray!
Identification as member of social group	Role	Formality of address	N (on phone): Good morning, Doctor, Nurse Burrows here.
	Shared knowledge	Talking 'shop'	N (to other N): . . . and then in the afternoon, they both took her to theatre.
		Using jargon	Sister: Nurse, did you say the BP for No. 6 was 110 over 90?
		Restricted codes	
Personal identity	Character	Personal anecdotes	P: I always went for a walk after church on Sundays
	Interests	Self-disclosure	N: When I were a li'l'un, I'ad some braw times wi' me da.
			N: I think canoeing sounds really interesting.
	Values and attitudes	Lies	P (to N): I had a cat that got run over once, too.
	Interpersonal attitudes		N: Oh, I hate just sitting quietly and reading.
			P: I need to go to the little boy's room.

Control/manipulation (1)	Interpersonal attitudes	Flattery	Junior Dr (*to student N*): You *do* do dressings well!
			N: Oh you've washed your hair – it does look nice!
		Tact	
		Compliments	
Control/manipulation (2)	Encounter regulations	Greetings	P: Hello, and how are you today after your break?
		Partings	N: It's nice to see you looking so well. 'Bye!
		Questioning { closed / open / leading	P: What do you think of it?
			N: Mm . . . Go on . . . .
			N: So you would like more information?
		Encouraging	
		Reflecting	
Control/manipulation (3)	Regulation of others' a) behaviour b) feelings	Instructions	N: Take both these pills now!
		Commands	N: Turn over!
		Requests	N: Please will you keep a record of the fluids you take today?
		Threats	P: If you do that again, I'm walking out.
		Jibes/jokes	N: You look like a chip waiting for vinegar!
		Reassurance	N: It's quite normal to feel upset.
Instrumental	Getting or achieving something	Requests	P: Will you let me go to the day room now?
		Hints	P: I am going to burst any minute.

Table 3.1 *Continued*

Function	Focus	Strategies	Examples
Rewardingness/interest as interaction partner	Character	Colourful speech	N (*to other N*): It was so fantastic – the heather was vivid and fragrant and the moss as springy as fresh-cut hay.
	Interests	Humour	P (*to N*): Another injection? No, I don't mind, they don't call me pop-a-bubble Peter for nothing!
Representational	Inform other role	Give information	N: Go up the corridor and take the first on the right.
		Answer requests	N: It will hurt at the time, but it should only last 3 – 4 hours.
			Dr: It's just a little test to see if the nerves are damaged.
Investigate	Acquire information to learn role	Questioning	P: What does D&C stand for?
			N: Have you been in hospital before?
Expressive	Personal identity	Exclamations	P: I hate sago!
	Emotional state	Swearing	P: You stick that bleedin' thing in me again . . .!
		Terms of endearment	N (*to child*): Come on, lovey . . . .

Escapism	Role Interpersonal attitude	Blocking Changing the subject	N: How are you feeling, OK? N: How soon will you recover? … What did you have for dinner?
	Personal identity	Joking	P: I'll say hello to St Peter at the Pearly Gates for you.
		False reassurance	N: Oh come now, there's no need to worry!
		Leading questions	N: That didn't hurt, did it?
Non-verbal accompaniment	Behaviour	Promising	N: I promise I'll come and see you later.
	Acts	Betting	P: I bet you I'll eat it all today.
Descriptions	Statements about the world	Stating	P: The floor needs cleaning.
		Reporting	N (to Sister): Mrs Perkins had a good night.
Social functions that are not primarily interpersonal Regulation of own			
a) behaviour	Self-control	Self-statements	N: Now, 250 cl dextrose …
b) feelings	Self-reassurance		P: Pull yourself together, it won't be that bad!
Aesthetics	Literature Poetry Messages	Creative speech/writing	e.g., poem written to N by grateful P.

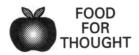

**FOOD
FOR
THOUGHT**

Which functions of speech are the most common in nurse-patient interactions? Why is this?

Which are the most common functions of speech fulfilled by patients? Why is this?

Do doctor-nurse interactions reveal some functions of speech more than others? Which ones?

Are there any functions of speech that are rare in nursing settings? Why might this be?

Are different functions of speech emphasised in community nursing from hospital nursing? Why?

as the **interaction context** in order to decide how to act appropriately (usually in order to achieve some social goal). It will often be necessary to look at an interaction over a period of time, in order to judge whether or not a particular strategy was effective. Examining speech, comment by comment, will not always tell us. Sometimes we may not even know whether a particular strategy was effective or not until we meet again on another occasion. So, for example, we may not know whether what we hoped would be reassuring was so until we meet again and are in a position to assess our partner's anxiety/concern over the issue; if s/he is still anxious at a later date, we may assume our 'reassuring' strategy has been ineffective. This raises an interesting question of how short- or long-term our strategies are or should be. There is probably no answer to this!

SUMMARY

This chapter has been concerned with verbal and non-verbal elements of social behaviour. Specifically, the following issues were raised:

- Non-verbal communication and speech interrelate in complex ways.
- Non-verbal cues form the bases of impressions of other people's values, attitudes, personality and interests.
- The meaning of social behaviour is linked to expectations stemming from the cultural and situational contest in which it occurred.
- Habits are learnt, convey little meaning and are difficult to change.
- Non-verbal communication is vital to the regulation of encounters.

- Dominance is achieved through the use of certain nonverbal behaviours.
- There are latent and manifest meanings in speech.
- Rules of conversation vary with culture and situation.
- Breaking rules of conversation may be meaningful.
- The context contributes to understanding of conversations.
- Regular patterns of speech, bound by rules, are called rituals.
- Rituals of speech occur in both formal and informal situations.
- Strategies of speech vary with role.
- Elaborated and restricted styles of speech have different social consequences.
- Language style both reflects and creates social relationships.
- The value of particular strategies of speech may be assessed from social reactions to them.
- Interaction contexts dictate which strategies of speech will be most effective.

SELF-DEVELOPMENT EXERCISES

1. Turn the sound down while you are watching television. How easy is it to know what the person talking is a) talking about b) thinking and c) feeling? Do you like the person talking? Why?
2. Sit with your back to the television. How easy is it to know what the person talking is a) talking about, b) thinking and c) feeling. Do you like the person talking? Why?
3. Think about your own non-verbal behaviour. During a conversation, try to change any two of your non-verbal behaviours. What effect does this have on your conversation and on other people's reactions? How easy was it to do this? What makes it hard?
4. Identify some of your own non-verbal or speech habits. Do they have any effect on other people? How do you know?
5. Identify three examples of nurse–patient conversation that have both latent and manifest meaning. How are misunderstandings due to level of meaning resolved?
6. Identify the rules of conversation in the following nursing situations: explaining a poor prognosis to a patient; making a primary assessment of a patient; giving infant nutrition advice to a mother in her own home; as a staff nurse, explaining to the Ward Manager the purpose of a small research project you would like to carry out on her/his ward; advising a colleague what to do about her/his career progression; talking with a GP about an elderly relative's future care; a ward round; a care conference. What happens if these rules are broken?

7. What conversation rituals can you identify in your nursing practice? What would happen if these rituals were not performed?
8. Identify four examples of restricted codes used by different health professionals in the course of one week. What is the impact of using restricted code?

CHAPTER 4

Social perception

Interpersonal skill is not only concerned with what we say or do; it is equally concerned with how astute we are in observing what other people say and do, and how we interpret what we notice (Markus and Zajonc, 1985). This sounds easy: either someone says/does something, or s/he does not. The problem is, though, that most people say and do far too much for us to notice and remember accurately everything that really happened. In fact, in our everyday lives we are extremely selective in what we notice about other people (Wegner and Vallacher, 1977). We make all sorts of judgements about others on the basis of a limited amount of factual information. As we grow up, we develop cognitive or mental frameworks that help us organize, interpret and remember that plethora of social information available to us in any situation. These frameworks are known as **schemata** (Fiske and Taylor, 1984). We form schemata from what we know about ourselves and other people, and from our general experience with life (Leyens and Codol, 1988). Once formed, the schemata determine both the ease with which new social information is processed and the efficiency with which it is brought to mind (Figure 4.1).

Our schemata encourage us to be extremely selective in what we perceive of other people's behaviour. While our schemata are formed on the basis of past experience, they can lead to distortions or biases in what we perceive (Hewstone and Antaki, 1988). For a start, we only attend to certain things and not to others. Often, those things we notice are of particular relevance to us for one reason or another. In other words, they fit in with our own 'construct systems' (Bannister and Fransella, 1980).

Sometimes we even make up things that we think are happening but are not: we **construct** social events. Having only attended to certain things, we may make errors in explaining or interpreting what we have observed (Niven, 1989). If these events have taken place some time previously, we **reconstruct** social events. In doing this, we remember some things and then assume certain other things (must have) happened as well. We generalize from one thing to another.

Many of these biases in person perception are due to the expectations we hold about what should (and what did) happen.

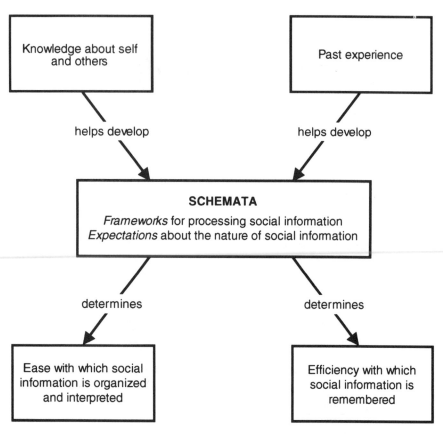

Figure 4.1 Development and functions of schemata in social perception (from Kagan, Evans and Kay, 1986).

Consider, for example, a qualified experienced nurse, a student nurse and a member of the public all entering an unfamiliar ward. They will all notice different things about the nurses working on the ward. Their past experiences will have led to the formation of different cognitive schema, construct systems and expectations about how the nurses are behaving. So, if they find all the nurses wearing jogging pants and T-shirts, the lay person may not even notice them, the student may be bemused but assume this ward permits such a thing and the experienced nurse may judge every-thing the nurses do as too sloppy or informal.

In this situation the lay visitor may have been more intent on finding the friend she came to visit than interested in the nurses. The experienced nurse may be proud of the formal standards she upholds in her own practice and the student may be open to new experiences. What each of them notices is of personal relevance and the interactions they make also depend on their different cognitive schemata.

The experienced nurse may retell this incident later on. She may assume that all the nurses were dressed informally when in fact only some of them were. On relating the incident later, the student may relate how informal the mealtimes were, when he did not actually see a mealtime. He generalizes from what he did see and his assumption of the permissive regime to other parts of the ward routine.

We will consider some major sources of error in perceiving other people.

LABELLING

When we hold expectations about other people's behaviour, attitudes, beliefs, character, etc. by virtue of the role they play, labelling may occur (Wegner and Vallacher, 1977; Stockwell, 1972). The labelling process is as follows:

Diagram 4a

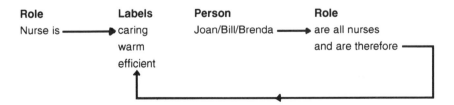

We expect that the **person** will possess the characteristics associated with the **role**. If these expectations are widely held, the person becomes 'labelled' and may find it very difficult not to adopt those characteristics. Wegner and Vallacher (1977, p. 105) say: 'even if a labelled person is not influenced by our expectation, we may still **think** that he or she is behaving as anticipated. . . . Once someone has been labelled, all his subsequent behaviours, even inconsequential ones, are interpreted in terms of that label.'

Stockwell (1972) drew attention to this process with reference to patients who were labelled 'unpopular'. A request from a demanding patient is not interpreted in the same way as a request from a patient who is usually no 'bother'.

Labelling may result in a **self-fulfilling prophecy** (Rosenthal and Jacobson, 1968) (that is, if we expect things to happen, they will) and is linked to the existence of stereotypes.

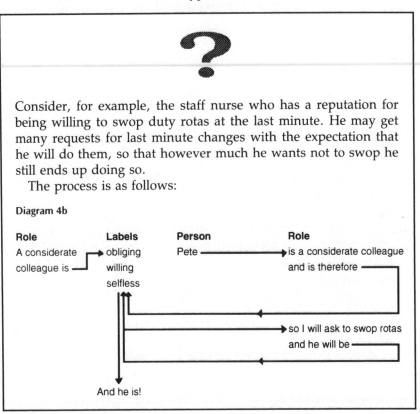

Consider, for example, the staff nurse who has a reputation for being willing to swop duty rotas at the last minute. He may get many requests for last minute changes with the expectation that he will do them, so that however much he wants not to swop he still ends up doing so.

The process is as follows:

Diagram 4b

Role	Labels	Person	Role
A considerate colleague is	obliging willing selfless	Pete	is a considerate colleague and is therefore
			so I will ask to swop rotas and he will be
	And he is!		

STEREOTYPES

Stereotypes are generalized statements about things. We all use stereotypes to help us organize and understand our social worlds. The process of stereotyping requires us to categorize things, attribute characteristics to the category and then infer that the things themselves possess those characteristics by virtue of belonging to the category (Forgas, 1985a, Wegner and Vallacher, 1977). We can hold stereotypes about people, objects, cultures, food, roles – anything in fact.

When we stereotype roles, there is a danger that this can lead to labelling and, in turn, to self-fulfilling prophecies. Some of the stereotypes we have are widely held, but others are more idiosyncratic and specific to ourselves. When these are concerned with the 'typical' characteristics different 'types' of people have, they are known as what Bruner and Tagiuri (1954) originally called 'implicit personality theories'.

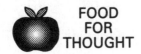

FOOD
FOR
THOUGHT

Where do a) patients b) relatives c) nurses get their expectations about each other from?

How do nurses' expectations affect patients?

Have you ever felt the influence of other people's expectations?

How much agreement between you and your friends would you expect in describing a) a typical irritating patient b) junior doctors c) interfering relatives? Where do the agreements or disagreements come from?

Are stereotypes ever useful? When?

What judgements do you and your friends make about other people's personalities, beliefs, attitudes, interests, styles of living and so on? What are these judgements based on?

What are the most important things you try to find out about someone when you first meet them? Why these things?

Have you ever employed implicit personality theories in your nursing career? When and how?

IMPLICIT PERSONALITY THEORIES

We all have ideas about the ways different types of people behave and why they do so. Forgas (1985a, p. 39) sums it up well when he says 'As a result of our accumulated knowledge about people, we all have an "implicit theory of personality", which may be defined as the sum total of our accumulated hypotheses and expectations about the way other people's attributes and traits are organized'. These theories are personal to ourselves and may not be shared by others. They arise primarily from our experiences of other people, our prejudices and our likes/

dislikes. However, we may have adopted certain beliefs about others from, for example, our parents: these may then be incorporated into our implicit personality theories.

We use our implicit theories of personality in order to make predictions (often wrongly) about how people we do not know very well behave, and thus how we should behave in relation to them. In forming impressions of people, Eiser (1980, 1986) suggests that we do so while explaining their behaviour. The attributions we make help impressions we have formed stick, and are, themselves, subject to a number of biases.

Our implicit personality theories are particularly important, as we have said above, when first meeting people. They help us form impressions of people which are generally hard to change. Having made judgements about people, we tend to regard everything they do in a light consistent with our initial judgements. Thus implicit personality theories too may lead to a self-fulfilling prophecy, through our desire to maintain consistency.

CONSISTENCY

In many different spheres of our social lives we seem to try to maintain consistency (Festinger, 1957). This is particularly so when we make social judgements. Although we like to think that they are not, first impressions can be resistant to change. We distort or explain away contradictory information so that we can maintain the consistency of our initial judgement. It has been suggested by Asch (1946) that we tend to group characteristics together, around the 'central traits' of **warm** and **cold**. Once we have judged people to be 'warm', or to possess some of the characteristics that are grouped around 'warm', we tend not to judge them as 'cold'. And of course, the converse also holds: having judged people to be 'cold', in order to maintain consistency in our judgements, we do not also see them as 'warm'.

Once we have made preliminary judgements about people in terms of their being warm or cold, our subsequent perceptions of them might be distorted as we strive to maintain consistency. A **halo effect** is said to operate (Forgas, O'Connor and Morris 1983). The danger here, again, is that the operation of the halo effect and maintenance of consistency in judgements about people may lead to a self-fulfilling prophecy. As Niven (1989, p. 55) puts it, 'patients who have created a positive impression on health staff will have their traits and abilities evaluated in a favourable manner, whereas those who, unfortunately, have not made such a good impression may, as a result of unfavourable evaluations, receive less interest and attention'.

PERSONAL RELEVANCE

At the beginning of this section, we mentioned that we are selective in what we notice about other people. What we perceive is influenced by our schemata: by our expectations, our stereotypes, our implicit personality theories and our need to maintain consistency. We will also perceive those things that have personal significance, especially those characteristics we can identify with and that we can judge to be similar to our own. Thus, when we meet someone who shares our values, attitudes or beliefs, or even a particular interest, we will judge him/her positively and attribute favourable characteristics to him/her. Furthermore, we may even generalize many of our own characteristics to him/her. This is another example of the halo effect at work. The distortions in perception that occur will be particularly strong if we share attitudes, values, beliefs and interests with the other person.

Consider, for example, the student nurse far from home who is overjoyed to find that the first patient she gets to know comes from her home town. The joy is increased if she finds they went to the same school. It will take this nurse a long time to recognize that she dislikes the patient. More importantly, though, she may jump at a false interpretation of the patient's distress, as she assumes they are so alike and understand each other so well. In this way a relationship may develop between them that is founded on false assumptions and contains many misperceptions.

Similar biases may emerge if we perceive the person as having characteristics dissimilar to our own. If we are fat, we may note immediately that our new acquaintance is painfully thin; others present for whom fat/thinness is irrelevant may not even notice. As before, selective perception, based on personal relevance, may lead to generalized expectancies and a self-fulfilling prophecy.

CONSTRUCTIVE AND RECONSTRUCTIVE SOCIAL PERCEPTION

We have seen in this section that 'accurate', 'objective' social perception is difficult to achieve. We construct our observations and interpretations of interpersonal events on the basis of the schemata we have developed over the years. Our expectations (based on past experience, anticipation of the future and present knowledge) encourage us to make unwarranted generalizations and to try to maintain consistency of judgement (Bartlett, 1932). As a result, much of what we 'perceive' to be the case may become a self-fulfilling prophecy, and turn out as expected. Similar biases are produced when we reconstruct our perceptions, based on (unreliable) memory. Eye-witness testimony is notoriously unreliable: so, too, is the evidence of our ears.

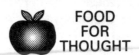

**FOOD
FOR
THOUGHT**

What sorts of things do you remember about people you have met briefly?
    What personal relevance do these have to you?
    Do you remember different kinds of things for people of different ages, sex and cultures? In what ways?

Our predisposition to construct and/or reconstruct our perceptions of other people can have serious consequences for our effective use of interpersonal skills in nursing. Perhaps the most crucial effect of the biases inherent in person perception is that they obscure us to the very individual nature of the other people we relate to. We are, in effect, 'blinded' to what other people are really doing and saying; this in turn may lead to the adoption of those behaviours, expressions of feelings, etc. that we have expected. In other words the self-fulfilling prophecy is realized and we thereafter assume that our initial perceptions were accurate! The process is illustrated in Figure 4.2.

It is important for us to bear in mind some of the sources of bias in person perception, and what our own tendencies to be consistent and/or to generalize are, if we are to begin to be able to make realistic observations, assessments and appraisals of our own interpersonal behaviour.

SUMMARY

This chapter has been concerned with the processes and biases underlying social perception. Specifically the following issues were raised:

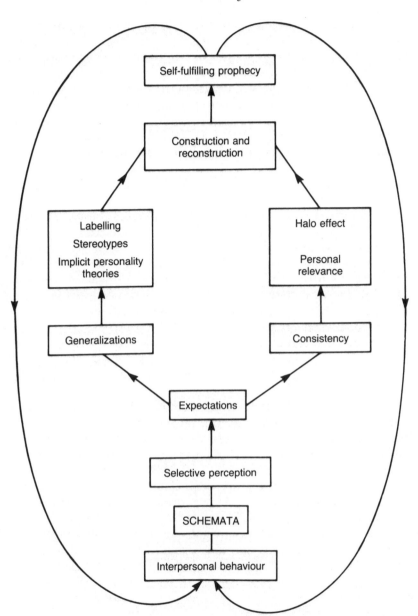

Figure 4.2 Social perception and the self-fulfilling prophecy (from Kagan, Evans and Kay, 1986).

- Perceptual aspects of interpersonal skill are as important as performance aspects.
- Observations about other people are selective, and interpretations of observations open to distortion.
- Schemata, or cognitive frameworks, develop that help us organize, interpret and remember social information.
- Schemata develop from our knowledge of self and others, from past experience.
- Schemata lead us to be selective in our perceptions and to hold expectations about what is happening.
- Expectations lead to the construction and reconstruction of social events.
- Expectations are the source of many different biases in social perception.
- Labelling may occur when expectations are held by virtue of another's role.
- Stereotyping may occur when expectations are held by virtue of categories of attributes.
- Expectations based on past experience may lead to the development of implicit personality theories.
- Most people attempt to maintain consistency between social judgements.
- First impressions are difficult to change, and may lead to a halo effect.
- Initial judgements about others frequently include either 'warm' or 'cold', which are thought to be central traits.
- Social judgements are often made on the basis of personal relevance.
- Expectations lead to the construction and reconstruction of social events, and this in turn may lead to the self-fulfilling prophecy.
- The self-fulfilling prophecy may lead to behaviours, or expressions of feelings, resulting from underlying expectations rather than from the person her/himself.
- Biases in social perception mitigate against one person treating another as an individual, and thus distort the effective use of interpersonal skills.

SELF-DEVELOPMENT EXERCISES

1. Take some time to talk to a colleague who works in a similar job to yours. When you both started the job, what pressures did you feel to carry it out in particular ways? Did you pick up that other people had particular expectations of you? Who did, and what were the expectations?

2. Identify the stereotype in each of the following scenarios:
   - The primary nurse for Sharon Smith, a 17-year-old with diabetes, comments: 'She's been admitted again, she's obviously not following her regime. Says she doesn't know how to test her blood sugar anyway, and doesn't want to. They're all the same these teenagers – too busy enjoying themselves to take responsibility.'
   - Mr Jones, aged 42, has just been admitted to the surgical ward. The nurse remarks: 'Well, what can you expect – he's a heavy drinker. Wouldn't be told about his alcohol consumption. It's no wonder his blood results are up the wall.'
   - At a care review, a district nurse says: 'Ethel is a sweet little lady who is doing quite well after her time in hospital after her fall at home. She's somewhat confused and forgets who we all are but considering she's 89 years old, she's surprising.'
   - Simon is a 19-year-old who discharges himself from psychiatric care regularly. The charge nurse comments: 'He really knows how to play the system. He's an angel when his Mum's here. He's terribly spoiled by his professional parents – used to being waited on hand and foot. It's no wonder he can't hold himself together.'
3. Discuss your impressions of someone you know slightly with a friend. To what extent do you agree on her/his character, personality, interests, abilities and so on? Upon what information or impressions are you basing your views? Where do you and your friend agree and disagree in your views about the other person? Why is this?
4. Think of two people you know who are quite different from each other. Jot down each of their qualities and characteristics. How many of them do the two people share and how many are quite different? Are there key characteristics you think distinguish different people? What are they? Do they apply to people from different cultural backgrounds?
5. Think of a recent time you and a friend went somewhere together. Discuss what you saw, heard and did with your friend. How much similarity in the detail you both gave was there? How might you decide who is correct and who is mistaken?
6. With five friends, play 'Chinese whispers'. One person gives a message and passes it on to the next, who passes it on to the next, and so on. The last person should repeat the message out loud. Discuss how similar or dissimilar the message is at the end from the one that began the game. Some possible messages are given below:
   - To get to the Out-Patients Department you need to walk about 200 yards down the main corridor. Keep watching for where the flooring changes to black and white tiles. Just after that you'll see a corridor on the right-hand side with a sign pointing to the Day

Hospital. Go downstairs and follow it as it winds up to the left. Go past the Occupational Therapy Department on your left and you'll see the Out-Patients Department entrance about 100 yards along at the end.

- You will need at least two litres of fluid a day, preferably water, though if you have soup or cups of tea, count these too. Keep on with the antibiotics eight-hourly for three days. In another week two tablets morning and evening. A week after finishing, let's have a midstream specimen of water – collect it first thing in the morning and put it immediately into this 30 ml sterile collecting bottle. Use the pessaries every night before you go to bed.

- When his mother calls, invite her in. Don't let her upstairs to his room – that's invasion of privacy. Make sure his shoelaces are done up and his zip is up. She will want to go as soon as possible so he will have to be ready. Make sure his coat is smart and on properly. Ask for money but be realistic – be prepared to say what it is for. He doesn't eat bread. Beer is OK but his mother won't think so.

CHAPTER 5

Social problem solving (1)

If we are to use interpersonal skills effectively, we have to be able to decide which to use in which situation. In other words, we have to think about what we want to achieve in a specific situation and choose an appropriate strategy. The ability to perceive social cues accurately and decide upon suitable social action is itself a skill, albeit a cognitive skill rather than a performance one (D'Zurilla and Nezu, 1982; Kagan, 1984). In this chapter we shall look at some cognitive aspects of inter-action. We will concentrate on social problem solving, with specific reference to the nature of attitudes and prejudice and attempts to change them.

THE SOCIAL PROBLEM-SOLVING PROCESS

Many interpersonal situations require that we think carefully of how we are going to handle them. In doing this, firstly we need to identify precisely what it is about the situation that is difficult or problematic. Following this, we need to think about alternative ways we could act and what the effects of these might be. Then, having chosen a course of action, we have to follow it, and finally attempt to assess whether we have, in fact, dealt with the problem effectively. Figure 5.1 summarizes the stages of social problem solving.

The skills that are part of social problem solving ability are, then:

- perception of social cues;
- accuracy in identifying own and others' goals;
- capacity to generate alternative strategies;
- the insight to judge the effectiveness of chosen strategies.

We have explored elsewhere (see Chapter 3) the perception of social cues.

The social problem-solving approach can be applied to any situation. It is not always as conscious as we have implied here: some people naturally adopt a problem-solving approach to various social situations. Indeed, it has been suggested that problem-solving ability distinguishes those who are rigid and relatively poor at dealing with interpersonal

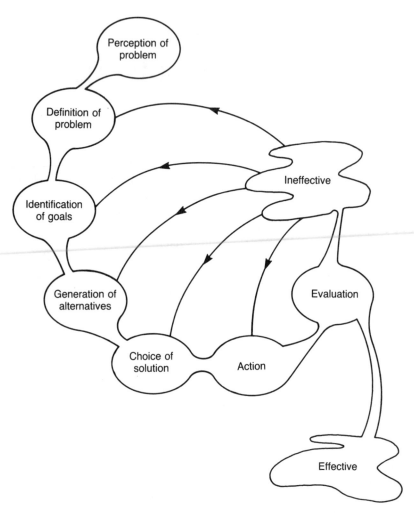

Figure 5.1 The social problem-solving process (from Kagan, Evans and Kay, 1986).

Consider, for example, a female medical ward in a large city general hospital. It is evening. Seven patients are in the day room after the visitors have left. Two Asian women are eating curried snacks brought to them by their visitors. A third Asian woman turns the TV on. A young white woman begins shouting (racial) abuse at the Asian women which attracts the attention of the ward Sister.

What should she do? And how should she go about it?

Perception of the situation: The Sister must notice that something is amiss and make judgements, from what she can see/hear, as to what is going on. As a result, she must **define the problem**. In the example, she may pick up what is being said and consider the problem to be either a dispute over choice of TV programme or a dislike of curry smells. On the other hand, she may consider the problem to be one of racial conflict. Her definition of the problem will lead her to think of possible outcomes or **goals**. She may, therefore, consider either a compromise over the TV programme, or the Asian women eating their snacks elsewhere, or a challenge to the white woman's racist views to be desirable goals, depending on her formulation of the problem. Having identified her goals, she must then consider various strategies she can use to achieve them. Once she has generated some alternative strategies, she must **choose** those that she thinks likely to be the most effective and then **act** on them. All the time she must be **evaluating** the current course of action to see if it is indeed effective. If it is not, she can do one of four things:

- reconsider the problem;
- change her objectives or goals;
- consider some alternative ways of achieving the goals;
- choose a different course of action.

From the moment she notices the disturbance, the Sister must run through, in her mind, the different stages of social problem solving, and change her behaviour accordingly until the problem is 'solved' to her satisfaction. Clearly, the better she is at doing this, the more effective she is likely to be.

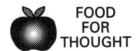

FOOD FOR THOUGHT

How easy is it to identify people's goals in social situations?

In a nursing situation are the patients' goals likely to be the same as the nurses'?

Once a social goal is identified, how easy is it to think of alternative strategies for achieving it?

Do our intentions in different nursing encounters change with a) the situation, b) the age of the person we are with and c) the cultural backgrounds of people involved? If so, how?

What cues do we use to predict what someone else wants out of a social situation?

Are any of the stages of problem solving more difficult than others? Which and when?

situations from those who are flexible and relatively adept at dealing with them (Kagan, 1981). It follows, then, that practice in social problem solving skills may lead to more effective interpersonal functioning (Hollin and Trower, 1986b; Trower, 1984).

The example we have given above is an interesting one in so far as it concerns not only people's behaviour but also their attitudes – in this case racist attitudes. As attitudes underlie a great deal of our interpersonal behaviour, and as nurses often try to get people to change their attitudes in one way or another, we will take some time now to discuss them.

ATTITUDES

Attitudes have no independent existence. So how do we know what people's attitudes are? Generally, we look at their behaviour and infer their attitudes from the way they behave (Fishbein and Ajzen, 1975). Stahlberg and Frey (1988) point out that attitudes will be weak predictors of behaviour when the situational constraints are so strong that little individual behaviour is possible. Similarly, it can be argued that we infer our own attitudes from seeing how we ourselves behave or perceive ourselves to be in control over our behaviour (Ajzen and Madden, 1986). One of the reasons we make judgements about other people's attitudes is so that we can make predictions about how they behave. Whilst this might appear sensible and a useful way of organizing a lot of information about others, it can lead us into difficulties as people do not always behave in accordance with their (assumed) attitudes (Fazio and Zanna, 1981).

The nature of attitudes

It can be useful to think of three parts of an attitude, as illustrated in Figure 5.2.

Firstly there is the cognitive or thinking part, for example, 'I think men and women are equally suited to nursing'. Then there is the affective or feeling part, for example, 'I feel angry when men are

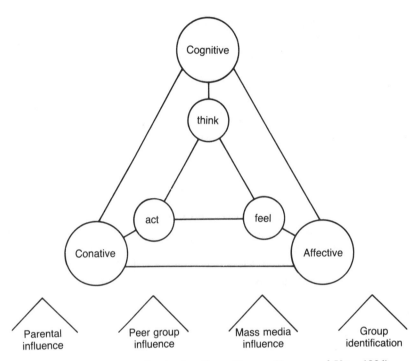

Figure 5.2 The nature of attitudes (from Kagan, Evans and Kay, 1986).

refused places on nurse training courses'. And finally there is the conative or action part, for example, 'I encourage men and women to apply for nurse training and do all I can to select suitable applicants whether they be men or women'. Rosenberg and Hovland (1960) first suggested this tripartite view of attitudes and the idea has been found to be useful ever since. It is generally assumed that the three parts of an attitude are consistent, but this is not always so and, as we shall see later, the inconsistency between parts of an attitude may be exploited in attempts to change attitudes (Cooper and Fazio, 1984).

So far, then, we have argued that attitudes are 'hypothetical constructs' in that they are inferred (sometimes inaccurately) from behaviour. It can be useful to think about the thinking, feeling and action parts of an attitude and the extent to which they are consistent with each other. Attitudes help us to make predictions about how we and others will behave and to express values about objects, events or people. These predictions may be about general social behaviour, or, importantly about health-related behaviour (Carter, 1990). As we can see from Figure 5.2 attitudes develop as a response to various influences, including parental/family, peer group, mass media or group identity influences. Social norms are, then, important determinants of attitudes. In other words, attitudes develop as part of the general process of socialization.

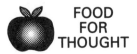

FOOD FOR THOUGHT

Where do your attitudes towards patients come from?

Is it more difficult to see where some attitudes have come from than others? Why is this?

Can you identify the most important socializing agent(s) for attitudes held by a) nurses and b) patients?

What role does a local health authority play in determining people's attitudes towards health?

How can we influence other people's attitudes?

What is the relationship between attitudes and professional interpersonal skills?

How might attempts to change patients' attitudes towards their own health-related behaviour be evaluated?

Sometimes attitudes can be particularly strong and lead us to have biased predictions about other people's behaviour. Such strong attitudes are known as prejudices, and if acted upon may amount to discrimination.

Prejudice

We are all prejudiced about some things, events or people.

Our prejudices are frequently based on stereotypes, are emotionally charged and, if they are expressed, take the form of discrimination. As such they have unpleasant interpersonal consequences. Unfortunately, prejudices are usually faulty, inflexible and difficult to change. One of the prerequisites for prejudice is that a person or an object can be seen to be different (and then discriminated against). Tajfel (1978) distinguished between interpersonal and intergroup behaviour. Interpersonal behaviour means acting as can individual whereas intergroup means acting as a member of a social group (behaving as a nurse, as a patient, as a man and so on). Prejudice may be an expression of either individual or intergroup behaviour; in both, the person or group towards whom the prejudice is directed is seen as different. This is one reason why racial prejudice is often linked with skin colour.

In nursing there are many opportunities to see other people as different, opportunities that are often linked with different illnesses or disabilities. Obvious examples are where there are clear signs and illness is easily detected. People with Parkinson's disease, facial palsy, scar tissue on face or hands, varying degrees of paralysis or spasticity, and those who are over/underweight, may all appear different, and thus be the objects of prejudice (Goffman, 1963). People with mental and physical disabilities, too, may be discriminated against as might those with degenerative diseases such as multiple sclerosis or motor neurone disease. People who need prostheses of one sort or another – ranging from glasses, hearing aids, tooth braces and neck supports to artificial limbs and aids such as sticks, frames or wheelchairs – can all be identified and stand in danger of being discriminated against.

Goffman (1963) discussed the role of stigma in social life. Stigma refers to the process whereby people are disqualified from full social acceptance because of some personal characteristic that marks them as different. This characteristic may be easily seen, such as physical or social impairments, or able to be concealed, such as some aspect of personal history. Their difference stigmatizes them and as a result they may be excluded from full social lives. The stigma forms part of the person's identity: similarly something that has introduced a stigma (such as illness or accident) may threaten a person's identity (Breakwell, 1986). The presence of a stigma causes tension for the person. This is either because the stigma is easily seen and the person is discredited as a result, or because it is not. For stigmata that can be concealed (the person is able to 'pass' in society) there is always the possibility that it will be discovered and the person will be discredited. Thus both a visible and an invisible stigma can cause considerable personal distress which, in the case of people who are ill, may exacerbate the distress they experience.

Consider, for example, the 72-year-old man with a colostomy. His friends do not know he has had one. There is no need for him to tell them. However, he may not want to go out for long periods of time 'in case the bag leaks'. His colostomy is a discreditable stigma – if it is 'discovered' people may think less of him. The fact that he may be discovered causes him some tension. Consider, too, the 42-year-old woman who cannot read. She may have developed strategies for coping which conceal her illiteracy from all those close to her, including her family. When she is admitted to hospital following an accident, her husband is asked to read

> her the meal choices as the ward is short-staffed and there is no
> one available to help her. This might be the first time he has
> found out she cannot read. Her stigma has changed from being
> a discreditable to a discredited stigma. Up until now she has
> been operating under what Egerton (1967) calls the 'cloak of
> competence'.

People will go to all sorts of lengths to disguise a lack of competence
and stigma. This may lead to social embarrassment or exclusion, and
health care staff need sensitive skills of assessment, sometimes, to
discover people's needs for assistance. Sometimes the 'cloak of competence' results in people not receiving services they need (Burton,
1991).

Behaviour, too, can be stigmatizing. Nurses are renowned for disliking (and possibly discriminating against) patients who ask a lot of
questions and generally play the 'patient role' contrary to expectations
(Roberts, 1984). Whatever the source of the prejudice that results in
discrimination, one of the ways to tackle it is by trying to change the
underlying attitudes.

Changing attitudes

We have said that looking at the three parts of an attitude can help us
plan methods of attitude change. Stroebe and Jonas (1988) discuss the
ways that our propensity to maintain consistency in many parts of our
lives is the key to attitude change. Taking the model of an attitude, a
change in any one part should result in changes in the others.

> Consider, for example, a hypertensive person who has been
> advised, as part of her/his treatment programme to cut salt out of
> her/his diet, but whose attitude remains one of scepticism to-
> wards the importance of diet in hypertension. Her/his negative
> attitude underlies her/his failure to follow the medical guidelines.
> The attitude is characterized by thoughts, feelings and actions
> that are all consistent with each other (for example, I **think** the
> role of diet is insignificant: I **dislike** the prospect of doing without

salt: I will carry on **using** salt). If we were able to create some inconsistency within this system, the attitude may change. So, for example, giving the patient information may change her/his thoughts: 'It seems the role of diet **is** significant, so I'll stop using salt and maybe it won't be so bad' (*change of attitude*). Alternatively, having the person in hospital may afford the chance to make her/him stop using salt, with a consequent change in the other components (hospital catering facilities permitting!) 'I have been forced to stop using salt, so there must be something in the link between diet and high blood pressure so I feel better about it' (*change of attitude*).

There are several different ways an attitude change can come about in whole or part, and we've illustrated only two. However, the principle remains – disrupt the consistency (or congruence or consonance as it is sometimes called) between components of an attitude and this will lead us to experience tension (or inconsistency, incongruence or dissonance) which we then try to remove by changing the other parts accordingly. This tension is called **cognitive dissonance**: it is thought to be unpleasant, and as a result we do all we can to reduce it. Of course, we may simply rationalize the change in the first part of the attitude (for example, 'the information I've been given is unreliable – hospital dieticians are unnecessarily ruthless', etc.), in which case no attitude change will follow. Walsh and Ford (1989) argue that change in nursing practice can be brought about by dissonance-creating strategies.

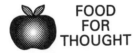 FOOD
FOR
THOUGHT

How easy is it to identify cognitive dissonance in people who are ill? How do nurses experience cognitive dissonance?

What strategies are used by a) patients, b) nurses and c) senior health professionals to reduce cognitive dissonance arising in work?

How might school nurses use cognitive dissonance to encourage school children to eat well?

How relevant are particular dissonance-creating strategies to people from different cultural backgrounds?

PERSUASION

There are many situations where nurses have to persuade other people to do something. Encouraging patient compliance with treatment regimes or health-related behaviour requires considerable understanding of what determines people's health-related behaviour, their knowledge of treatment as well as high levels of interpersonal skills. People's health beliefs (Becker *et al.*, 1979; Rosenstock, 1974, 1990), the information they have retained about their treatment (Inui and Carter, 1985; Ley, 1972, 1989) and the interpersonal skills of staff supporting them (Becker and Maiman, 1980; DiNicola and DiMatteo, 1982, 1984; DiMatteo and DiNicola, 1982) all influence degrees of compliance. Nurses may have to persuade patients about the advisability of doing certain things connected with their illness and/or treatment, or persuade colleagues to co-operate in some way. The issues at stake will vary from those about which nurses have little commitment to those about which they feel deeply concerned. Whatever the issue, though, persuasion must be planned and the social problem-solving process outlined above is a useful framework for thinking about effective persuasion (Figure 5.1).

Effective persuasive appeals

McGuire (1981) suggests a model of communication-behaviour change that can be incorporated into a social problem-solving process. In addition to the phases of social problem solving, three other factors must be considered. Firstly, the source of the persuasive appeal will affect how readily it is absorbed; so, conveying who it is that authorizes the message will influence its strength.

Consider, for example, various attempts to get people to change their diet or activities in the name of health education. If second-year student nurses were to endorse, say, the importance of taking more exercise for physical wellbeing, they would have little impact. If, however, senior physicians (in white coats!) or top sports personalities endorse the message, it may well have greater impact for certain groups. Thus the credibility, popularity and trustworthiness of the persuader should be considered.

Secondly, the nature of the communication – the message itself and the medium through which it is sent – will influence its acceptability. The message may be emotional or fear-producing and may or may not have specific recommendations for action. It may appeal to reason, presenting a one- or two-sided argument; it may be humorous and entertaining; it may contain the essence of the message at the beginning, middle or end of the total communication and it may or may not take into account the present level of opinion. The message may be spoken, written, recorded, drawn, videotaped or in the form of a song or play, and so on. Different messages to different audiences will require different types of persuasive appeals.

Finally, the nature of the audience or recipients of the communication must be considered. If people have had prior experience of attempts to be persuaded, they may have been 'inoculated' against the appeal, and thus react against further attempts at persuasion: furthermore, people with low self-esteem are more easily persuaded and *vice versa*. A group audience may react differently from individual(s) to different types of appeal. The factors to bear in mind when planning a persuasive message are summarized below.

Factors influencing persuasive appeals

Source (Who)
Credibility and expertise
Popularity (media/sports/pop stars, etc.)
Trustworthiness (related to triviality of issue)

Nature (How?)
1. Message:
    a) Emotionally arousing/appealing to reason
    b) One- or two-sided argument
    c) Order of presentation
    d) Present opinions of audience
2. Channel:
    a) visual
    b) auditory
    c) entertainment

Audience characteristics (to whom?)
Initial position

Level of self-esteem
Group/individual(s)
Prior experience and 'inoculation'

Effects (What should change?)
Behaviour
Attitudes
Thoughts

In short, persuasion must take account of who says what to whom *via* what medium and with what effect? This last point is an important one as, in order to gauge whether or not persuasion was effective, we should have some idea of what a desirable change would be (for example, a behaviour or attitude change). McGuire's (1981) model specifies a 12-step sequence if long-term behaviour change is to be achieved. The steps are:

1. exposure to the communication;
2. attending to it;
3. liking, becoming interested in it;
4. comprehending it (learning what);
5. skill acquisition (learning how);
6. yielding to it (attitude change);
7. memorizing it (content or agreement or both);
8. information search and retrieval;
9. deciding on basis of retrieval;
10. behaving in accord with decision;
11. reinforcement of desired acts;
12. post-behavioural consolidation (maintenance).

All persuasive attempts by nurses, whether in the context of health education or during the course of everyday nursing practice, can be judged against their 12 steps: have they all been incorporated?

Consider, for example, the school nurse working with a group of 15-year-old girls on the general topic of personal loving relationships, 'safe' sex and contraception. Giving information will not be enough to ensure attitudes and behaviours consistent with safe and responsible sexual relationships. The nurse must ask herself (and answer) the following questions in order to increase the effectiveness of her work.

- How will I present the issues in ways that will keep the girls' attention?
- How will I make it interesting and enjoyable?
- How will I ensure they learn the important facts?
- What behaviour do I want them to learn (and how will I help them do it in ways that are interesting and enjoyable?)
- How will I monitor and secure attitude change if necessary?
- What techniques will I use to help them remember?
- How will I help them retrieve important information when needed?
- How can I encourage and check on appropriate behaviour?
- How will I reinforce appropriate behaviour and make inappropriate behaviour less likely?
- How will I try to help them consolidate their learning when they are faced with difficult personal situations?

We can see that some interpersonal issues arise when these questions are asked. Most important are a) the timescale over which the activity takes place – in this case a long period of time is indicated – and b) the extent of trust and safety that is needed for the girls to talk quietly and honestly about their feelings and experiences.

Persuasion is often used in attempts to change attitudes and, in turn, to change behaviour, It can be argued that perhaps the greatest challenge to nurses is how to effect changes in their patients that require their willingness and co-operation. Medical and nursing procedures cannot always be imposed upon patients, and the interpersonal aspects of those procedures require nurses to have considerable social problem-solving skills.

SUMMARY

This chapter has been concerned with social problem-solving skills and their application in the context of attitude change and persuasion. Specifically the following issues were raised:

- Cognitive aspects are as important as performance aspects of interpersonal skill.
- Social problem-solving ability is fundamental to effective interpersonal skill.

- Perception of the situation leads to definition of the problem.
- It is necessary to identify the goals or possible outcomes before engaging upon a course of action.
- Appropriate strategies must be considered in pursuit of the identified goals.
- When a strategy has been chosen, it must be carefully monitored and evaluated to see if it is having the desired effect.
- On evaluating the effects of a particular strategy the options to change goals or reconsider alternatives should remain open.
- The more flexible a person is with regard to social problem solving, the more interpersonally skilled s/he is likely to be.
- The more rigid a person is with regard to social problem solving, the less interpersonally skilled s/he is likely to be.
- Social problem solving is not always a conscious process, but at any time it can become so.
- Attempting to change attitudes is a common social problem-solving situation for nurses.
- Attitudes do not exist, they are inferred.
- Attitudes can be thought of in terms of cognitive, emotional and behavioural components.
- A change in any one component may result in changes in other components.
- Inconsistency between parts of an attitude may lead to the experience of cognitive dissonance.
- People attempt to reduce cognitive dissonance whenever they can.
- Prejudice is a strong attitude and if acted upon may lead to discrimination.
- Prejudice and discrimination are closely linked to stigma.
- Stigma may be real or perceived.
- Prejudice is difficult to change.
- Persuasion is often used in attempts to change attitudes and/or behaviour.
- The source, nature and medium of the message all influence persuasive appeals.
- Audience characteristics influence persuasive appeals.
- Persuasion is a particular form of social problem solving.

SELF-DEVELOPMENT EXERCISES

1. Watch a film of some nursing activities (for example from a television documentary (such as *Jimmy's*) or drama (such as *Casualty*). See if you can identify the goals of any nurse at different points in time. Think what alternative strategies s/he could use to achieve the same goal, given the context in which s/he is working.

2. In the course of your work try to notice strategies that colleagues use to achieve particular goals. Do these strategies vary with profession, age, sex, culture or context? In what ways? Think of a tricky situation you successfully handled recently. What alternative ways might you have handled it? Think of a situation that did not work out as expected. Why was this? How might you handle a similar situation differently in future?

3. How might you deal with the following situations using a problem-solving approach?

   - You are the primary nurse looking after Ernest Jones (75 years old) who is thought to have a degenerative neurological condition. His progress and his prognosis is poor. Mrs Jones, his wife, has travelled a lengthy and difficult journey by public transport to keep an appointment with the senior house officer in order to discuss her husband's condition. She is herself quite severely disabled with osteoarthritis. As you see her approaching the ward door, looking tired and strained, the telephone rings: the doctor has to cancel the appointment to see Mrs Jones this evening.

   - You are working in the community and making a visit to Jane Fitzgerald, a woman living on her own with multiple sclerosis. While you are talking, there is a knock at the door, which is then opened from the outside with a key. It is Jane's sister, who enters directly into the living room where you are both seated. Jane is not pleased to see her and asks her to leave immediately, reminding her that they quarrelled fiercely last time they met. She also asks her to return the key and states firmly that she does not wish her sister to visit again.

4. With a friend, discuss your attitudes towards smokers, churchgoers, disposable hospital equipment, nurses who leave the profession and abortion. How did your attitudes come about? What was the influence of home, peers, school, groups with which you identify, your professional training and the media on the attitudes you hold?

5. Have you ever influenced anyone else's attitudes? How did you do this? How did you know you had this influence?

6. What prejudices do you hold? How did they develop? Are there any particular prejudices that create tension for you as a nurse?

7. What cognitive dissonance are the following likely to experience: people who are obese and unsuccessfully dieting; smokers who have no intention of giving up; a child with recurrent severe headaches who worries about the school she misses because of them? What dissonance-reducing strategies might each of them adopt? How might creating dissonance bring about change in nursing practice?

8. With two or more colleagues, prepare a persuasive appeal about one

of the following: having flu vaccine; using condoms for safe sex; attending breast screening or cervical cytology clinics; not bringing food on to hospital wards; preventing the closure of a mother and baby clinic; joining the Directorate nursing research interest group. How might you assess whether or not the appeal had been successful?

CHAPTER 6

Social routines

A great deal of social behaviour is predictable, following regular patterns. We have seen that the concept of 'ritual' is useful to describe regular patterns of speech based on a shared understanding of their meaning by both speaker and listener. The notion of social ritual, however, extends beyond speech to encompass regular patterns of complex social behaviour. In this section we shall examine the extent to which such patterns of behaviour are linked to the roles that people occupy and the rules they follow (Goffman, 1967).

SOCIAL ROLES

Drama and aspects of the theatre have provided a powerful metaphor for social behaviour. Erving Goffman (1959) developed a 'dramaturgical' approach to interaction, wherein people become actors playing roles and following scripts in different scenarios to different audiences, in other words what Harré and Secord (1972) call role–rule contexts. Just as actors play different parts in different plays, each with its own scenery, props and scripts, so people occupy roles in different situations, each with its setting, props and expectations held by all the people involved. Roles are, then, the parts we play or the behaviours that are expected from people who occupy different positions in different situations. The more formal the role, the more tightly scripted it is and the fewer the variations in behaviour associated with that role. Various pressures are brought to bear on people enacting their roles.

Firstly, the situation itself makes different demands on people occupying different positions (Argyle, Furnham and Graham, 1981). So the ward situation demands different behaviour from student nurses, ward sister, consultant, patients, visitors, etc. Sometimes these demands are made explicit via, for instance, ward regulations for all to see, such as 'No visitors to enter the ward until the screen is removed'. Sometimes they are implicit and conveyed by word of mouth or just assumed, such as that patients should not talk to Doctors on their ward round. The less clearly stated the demand, the more scope there is for people to express their roles in their own fashion, but also the more likelihood there is that they will make 'mistakes' and behave inappropriately.

Secondly, the expectations we and others have regarding how those in given positions should behave create pressures to learn appropriate behaviour (Milgram, 1974; Stone and Faberman, 1970). The stronger these expectations – or the stronger we believe them to be – the greater the pressure. Again, the more explicit the expectations, the less likelihood there is that inappropriate behaviour will develop.

The third influence is that wielded by the role partner: in order to give meaning to a role, there must be a complementary role. So for the role of 'nurse' to be meaningful, there must be patients/doctors/social workers, and so on. The ways our role partners act towards us and expect us to behave help us behave appropriately in our role. Thus we can see that roles are defined and constrained by (sets of) expectations.

Role conflict

Whenever there is conflict between one (set of) expectation(s) and another, we experience role conflict (Gahagan, 1984) and this can have repercussions for both how we behave and how we feel. Examples of role strain/conflict are shown in Figure 6.1.

Whenever we experience role conflict or strain, we try to resolve it in some way in order to reduce it. The social system itself often provides a means of coming to terms with the competing expectations of role partners and the demands of new situations.

Consider, for example, the ways in which further professional training helps ease hospital nurses into new roles in the community. Part of this training enables the future community nurses to discover other people's expectations of them and how these fit in with their own interpretation of the role. If community placements take place early in the course the students are quickly placed into positions of responsibility and they may experience role strain. The situation is made more difficult as the important role partners – patients – often expect the students to know everything. They will not always distinguish between 'community nurse' and 'hospital nurse trying to work in the community'. The students may feel pressure to act as if they are competent community nurses, or to tell the patients that they are in training. Either course of action could relieve the role strain or increase it.

Placements later on in the course evoke less role strain because students are by then, more accustomed or reconciled to their roles.

When we experience conflict through multiple role occupancy, the way to resolve it is to prioritize roles. A further method we have of resolving role conflict is to take some personal action. The nurse who feels conflict at being asked to do something s/he morally disagrees

1. Different expectations or lack of agreement amongst role partners, e.g. General Practitioner wants CPN to make regular visits to patient to monitor deterioration in mental health; Patient does not want CPN to visit; Psychiatrist wants CPN to get patient to attend outpatient clinic.

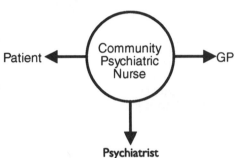

2. Different expectations or lack of agreement between role partners, e.g. Patient expects District Nurse to make her a cup of tea when she arrives (a); Nurse expects Patient to make her own tea (b).

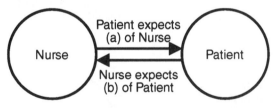

3. Personal expectations differ from situational demands.

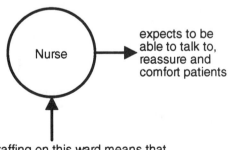

Figure 6.1 Role strain (adapted from Kagan, Evans and Kay, 1986).

4. Expectations from role
   partners clash with
   own principles

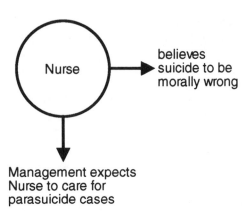

5. Lack of clarity in
   situational demands

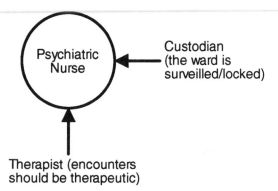

6. Personal characteristics
   unable to fulfil
   expectations

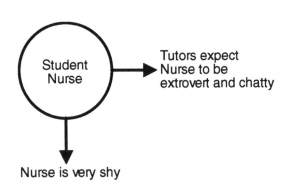

Figure 6.1 *Continued*

7. Multiple occupancy

Ann is Doris and Harold's daughter. Her parents place expectations on her which she tries to fulfil.

Ann becomes a Nurse and has demands made on her by patients, doctors and colleagues

Ann marries Kevin. He makes demands on her as his wife.

What will Ann do when her mother is admitted to the ward on which she works just as she is about to go off duty, having arranged with her husband to go out that evening? ...*crisis*

Note: Arrows pointing towards circles signify demands (usually external)
Arrows pointing away from circles signify expectations (usually internal)

Figure 6.1 *Continued*

with may either rationalize her/his situation or may opt out of the strained role altogether. There is quite a bit of evidence to suggest that one of the reasons why student nurses leave the profession is because of the conflict they experience between the reality of the demands made on them as nurses, and what they perceive the public's expectations of them as nurses to be. Role strain and conflict can become a source of stress and may lead to dissatisfaction with the job or burnout (Dolan, 1987; Lindop, 1989).

We have seen that roles are defined by sets of expectations that we, and others, have of the appropriate behaviours associated with them. These expectations may lead to the experience of role strain or conflict which we try to resolve in various ways. The expectations come from ourselves as individuals, the groups to which we belong, the organizations in which we work or even from the wider social/cultural context in which we live. They are transmitted by norms or social rules, which we learn via the process of socialization (Gergen, 1985).

NORMS AND SOCIAL RULES

Norms and social rules influence both the expression of roles and the expectations surrounding them. Given a particular role, the norms or rules give some guidance as to how it should be expressed. Thus roles and rules are closely linked, and together form what is known as the role–rule context of interpersonal behaviour (Harré and Secord, 1972; Marsh, Rosser and Harré, 1978).

The efficacy of interpersonal skills is inextricably linked to role–rule

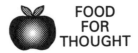 FOOD
FOR
THOUGHT

How much of your behaviour is linked to your role of nurse? Does this depend on the situation you are in? In what ways?

Are there any times you feel particular loyalty to the nursing profession, your school of nursing, or the team you work in? What makes you feel like this?

What are the norms of a) nursing and b) your health care team? How do you know?

In what circumstances do norms cease to guide people's behaviour? Has this ever happened to you?

contexts (Argyle, 1986; Trower, 1984). The acquisition of good inter-personal skill necessitates an appreciation of the nature of different role–rule systems in order to know how to behave and how to inter-pret other people's behaviour. Furthermore, once we understand the extent to which role–rule systems define and constrain our inter-actions, we can begin to see that the use of good interpersonal skills is not only restricted by the people displaying those skills, but is in part determined by the culture, the situation and other people's expec-tations (Harré, 1979; Burton, 1985; Lillie, 1985). In other words, inter-personal skill is not to be seen in isolation from the social system: instead, it is just one facet of interpersonal behaviour and is subject to many influences. (This theme will be developed further in Chapter 15.) We saw (Chapter 4) that strong expectations can result in self-fulfilling prophecies, whereby people may adopt the behaviours expected of them.

The identification of those specific norms that guide individuals and/or groups may help us to understand some of the (sub)cultural variations in social behaviour, and adjust our own perceptions and/or behaviour accordingly (Bochner, 1981).

The recognition that norms exist may help us understand some of the regular patterns of behaviour that are associated with both roles and situations. Furthermore, the consequences of either not behaving according to norms or deliberately breaking the rules are often in terms of the effect this has on interpersonal skills and relationships.

SOCIAL RITUAL

Social rules form the basis of the regular patterns of behaviour that occur in interpersonal situations and that vary with the role. Goffman (1967, 1971) describes many of these interpersonal exchanges as 'inter-action rituals'. These rituals may occur frequently and in different situations and appear to lose their surface (or manifest) meaning. However they do serve important social functions. Goffman suggests that they are essential for maintaining relationships and thus enabling social interaction to continue over time. He describes two sorts of rituals which serve this function: **supportive rituals** confirm the relation-ships in what he called good states of repair (greetings, farewells etc.) and **remedial rituals** repair those relationships that stand in danger of breaking down (apologies, excuses, etc.).

The supportive rituals of greetings and farewells, or introduction openings and closures, have received a lot of attention.

Openings and closures are of a special significance because of their potential for impact on the quality of the encounter: if we 'get off on the wrong foot' the entire interaction may be counterproductive, and if we 'end on a sour note' further interactions may be jeopardized. Generally, openings and closures are highly structured, containing large elements of ritualized behaviours, and are common to many different (sub)cultures.

Interaction openings

The tone of an interaction is usually set by the way it is opened. Hargie, Saunders and Dixon (1981) refers to the skills of the 'set induction' ('set' refers to the state of readiness or expectation that people are in; 'set induction' is the ways people can be prepared for the encounter to follow). An opening involves far more than just the words that are spoken. All the non-verbal cues expressed by each person help to give the others an idea about what is to follow.

Consider, for example, the community psychiatric nurse who is visiting the relatives of Roger, a young man who was admitted to hospital against his will earlier in the day. If she walks slowly up the path and looks down when the door is opened, she creates an expectation in the relatives about what she is about to say. They may well prepare themselves for bad news and might be somewhat bemused if she tells them brightly that Roger has settled down happily in the hospital and realizes he needs to be there.

A particular 'set' was created that was inconsistent with the nature of the interaction that followed.

The physical setting of an encounter may also lead people to have expectations about what is to follow. A patient who finds floor cushions rather than chairs in the clinic when s/he attends as an orthopaedic outpatient, may behave (and expect others to behave) in an unusual fashion.

What is actually said in greeting, or in opening conversation, is of crucial importance and tells each participant a great deal about how the other perceives their relationship and expects the interaction to proceed. For the more task-related interactions, the opening may include an attempt by one (or even both) partner to discover the extent to which the other knows about the task to be undertaken.

Consider, for example, the community nurse who is helping staff, who work with Jean, a 35-year-old woman with severe learning disabilities, to teach her to pour hot liquids. Before he outlines the backward chaining programme he has designed, he may first try to find out what the staff know about behavioural techniques in general and behavioural chaining in particular. This will help him decide how and what to tell the staff about the introduction of the programme.

Table 6.1 Functions of interaction openings

Social functions	*Task or cognitive functions*
Attracting and gaining attention	Ascertaining the extent of
Expressing relationships/roles	knowledge held about the
Establishing rapport	topic or the purpose of the
Arousing the motivation/ interest of a	encounter
partner	Indicating the objectives of the
Ascertaining others' expectations	encounter
Indicating the purpose of the encounter	Explaining one's functions and
Establishing links with previous encounters	limitations

Broadly, the functions of interaction openings are as shown in Table 6.1.

How could each of these functions be fulfilled? Many opening sequences serve several functions at once.

Interaction closures

Our feelings of satisfaction with an encounter, liking for our partners, sense of achievement and expectations for future meetings are affected by the way the interaction is closed. Hargie, Saunders and Dixon (1981) refer to closures as 'set closures' and discuss a number of ways of ending conversations so that relationships stay positive and the way is clear for further encounters in the future. As with openings, closures involve both non-verbal and verbal behaviours. Closures can include sequences or episodes of behaviour, and need not be restricted to relatively short parting statements. Different situations require different styles of closure. When a lot of information has been exchanged, closures may be used by either party to summarize or clarify the material that has been covered. If the encounter was highly emotional, as for example in a counselling interaction, closure may be used to 'wind down' so as to finish the session effectively. In such circumstances, closure can take quite a lot of the total time of the session. If either person is left feeling dissatisfied in any way at the end of the interaction, this can severely affect how s/he approaches future meetings. An unsatisfactory set closure may contribute to an unsatisfactory set induction prior to the next meeting. It is important, therefore, to have a clear idea of how we want to leave the interaction, and to possess the skills to put this into practice.

Consider, for example, the nurse who has been talking to Mrs Briggs, who has recently had a tumour removed from her duodenum. Mrs Briggs has been exploring the possible reasons for the tumour. The nurse has been listening sympathetically and pointing out the irrationality of some of Mrs Briggs's ideas. Suddenly the nurse jumps up, saying 'Ah well, nine o'clock, end of shift, time I was off. 'Bye', and leaves. Mrs Briggs may well feel that she has been a nuisance and silly; she probably won't want to discuss things with that nurse again.

Often, when we have informal conversations we end them by making excuses, such as 'I must go and see how Mrs Tompkins is getting on', rather than by saying something socially supportive such as 'I've enjoyed our talk – thanks. Perhaps we can continue it tomorrow?'

If one of the functions of set closures is to prepare for the next meeting, the latter strategy will be more effective than the former.

The functions of interaction closures are shown in Table 6.2.

How could each of these functions be fulfilled? Some of the strategies that can be used in closures are similar to those in openings. The use of open questions can discover whether the information reported has been taken in, or whether our partner has some 'unfinished business' (usually of an emotional nature) that should be dealt with.

If we want to leave the situation in a positive way, we should generally try to end on a supportive note. So, for example, a patient who has just co-operated with a painful procedure, such as a lumbar puncture, may be told 'You did very well, there. It's not easy having

Table 6.2 Functions of interaction closures

Social functions	Task or cognitive functions
Encouraging a sense of achievement	Indicating topic is completed (for the moment)
Indicating each other's degree of satisfaction and enjoyment	Focusing attention on essential material covered
Maintaining interest for future encounters	Assisting in consolidating facts, skills, concepts, arguments
Dissipating any agitation that had been aroused	Ascertaining whether the objectives of the encounter have been fulfilled
Communicating interpersonal attitudes	Indicating future courses of action
Indicating nature of future encounters	
Establishing the possibility that rapport is likely in the future	
Terminating attention	

that done. You really were helpful,' in a convincing way. These task-related comments may then be followed by some socially supportive comment, such as 'How do you feel now it's over?' This will only be valuable if full attention is paid to the reply, and the question is not asked in an accusing way that is really saying 'Don't you dare say anything other than "OK"'!

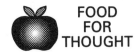

**FOOD
FOR
THOUGHT**

What is the relative importance of physical setting, non-verbal behaviour and speech for effective interaction openings and closures?

What variety of set inductions and closures do you use? What different functions do they serve?

To what extent do role–rule contexts determine interaction openings and closures?

How easy is it to 'recover' from misunderstood or badly handled interaction openings and closures?

Do people of different ages, sexes or cultural groups respond differently to interaction openings and closures?

What different set induction and closures would you use for: a) children; b) people who are aggressive; c) people who do not speak English; d) people you are visiting for the first time in their own home; e) an old friend you haven't seen for a long time?

As with openings, closures will usually fulfil more than one function at a time.

Remedial rituals

There are a number of rituals associated with repairing relationships – clearing up misunderstandings or overcoming mistakes. Again, while these exchanges may have ceased to have manifest meaning, they have important social functions, largely associated with keeping informal as well as working relationships positive. If relationships that have been damaged are repaired badly or clumsily, things can get worse instead of better.

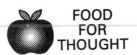

FOOD FOR THOUGHT

How do you know what kinds of apologies will be acceptable in different situations?

Are there cultural differences in ways of excusing or complaining of behaviour that has been inappropriate? What are they?

What are the differences in remedial exchanges made by women, men and children? Are any of these more effective than others?

Skill is required to repair relationships in ways that are genuine and do not appear to tokenistic or defensive.

Consider, for example, the nurse who leaves 83-year-old Mrs Roberts calling for a bedpan, saying 'With you in a tick!' Fifteen minutes later she returns, saying 'Crikey, I forgot!' and rushes off to get the pan. Another five minutes later she returns with the pan and says 'Doris is upset again' or 'We're rushed off our feet today' or 'There, you didn't mind waiting, did you?' She may well find Mrs Roberts snappy and rude and refusing to answer questions or have a conversation. Mrs Roberts may well 'go into a huff' with that nurse for several days.

> The danger with this kind of situation is that Mrs Roberts may be called uncooperative and sullen, when what has happened is a failure to repair a damaged relationship. How might this situation have been repaired more effectively?

FUNCTIONS OF SOCIAL ROUTINES

Interaction openings and closures are examples of ritualized social routines. They vary with the situation, the role of the participants and wider social cultural factors, such as the nationality, age, sex and social class of the participants. Different (sub)cultures and situations have different rules associated with them that prescribe appropriate behaviours. Nevertheless, such routines and rituals help us know how to behave and how to interpret other people's behaviour.

What we must remember is that our own behaviour, too, is likely to be interpreted according to other people's appreciation of the nature of social rules. This may result in a breakdown in social relations that we had not anticipated. The other important thing to note is that interpersonal skill (or lack of it) does not simply reside in ourselves as individuals. Much of our behaviour is constrained by what is expected of us in fulfilling our roles in particular situations. We must be aware of this if we are to plan effective use of interpersonal skills.

TRANSACTIONAL ANALYSIS

We have said above that the concept of role is part of a dramaturgical approach to social behaviour. Goffman suggests that in much of the ritualized behaviour, people (the **actors**) follow **scripts**. Sometimes the same scripts are used on different occasions when familiar **performances** are given or similar expectations are exerted by different **audiences**. Harré and Secord (1972) draw attention to the fact that very formal roles and rituals have scripts that are written down and followed closely (for example priests officiating at weddings, policemen issuing people with their rights on arrest).

Scripts are also central to another very different approach to social interactions and social routines which also uses the metaphor of drama, namely Transactional Analysis (Berne, 1964, 1973).

Scripts

Not only do people and families have scripts that they follow, but organizations and the subcultures within them do too (Jongeward, 1976). 'Organizational scripts include the institutionalized injunctions and permissions regarding expectations from all levels of employment in (and) in about such things as sex roles, grooming and dress, personal conduct, and working hours' (Jongeward and James, 1981, p. 9).

The scripts that people and organizations follow affect health care as they guide the perceptions, experiences and treatment of health sickness. If we can become aware of the patterns created by different kinds of scripts we can either follow them or try to rewrite them so that they are more constructive.

Ego states

Berne suggests that people retain as adults three ego states which can be separate and distinct sources of behaviour: the Parent ego state, the Adult ego state and the Child ego state. Although the Parent, Adult and Child are present in all of us, at any time one may be more 'charged' than others.

Consider, for example, the patient who comes for investigatory tests. He is worried and fearful (Child). The nurse tries to allay his fears by reassuring him (Parent). As the patient consults his diary to check dates for a follow-up appointment he thinks through the time other commitments may take (Adult).

Parent ego states contain the attitudes and behaviours internalized from outside sources, especially parents, church, school, professional training. Parent ego states express either critical, judgemental behaviour or mothering, supportive behaviour.

Adult ego states are oriented to reality and rational gathering of information and thought. The adult organizes, adapts, thinks things through and makes decisions.

Child ego states contain impulses that come naturally to infants. They can be volatile and uninhibited, showing emotions and reactions very easily.

In many ways the ego states are like roles. The idea is that we can look at transactions (or exchanges) between people in terms of the roles they adopt in relation to each other (Adult–Child; Adult–Adult; Parent–Child, etc.).

We often develop patterns of behaviour linked to our ego states, scripts and partners. Sometimes we may get stuck in these patterns and our behaviour becomes unrealistic, but with social consequences as we discussed above. Sometimes these rituals are characteristic of the particular people ('Oh, oh, here we go again, Richard putting everyone down (critical Parent) as usual'); or characteristic of particular situations (at the same time every day the nurse says 'The dinner has arrived, please will you sit at the table now' (Adult)); or characteristic of particular interactions ('Let's just watch Mark wind Peter up as usual (Child) and Peter get defensive (Child)').

By understanding the nature of interactions as expression of different ego states, it is possible to see how misunderstandings arise or when things go smoothly. It is possible to describe transactions as complementary (a message from one ego state gets the expected

Consider, for example, the community nurse at a care planning conference, who says 'Here is Miss Edwards's medical report' (Adult to Adult), only to be greeted by the social worker's reply, 'Does it always take you this long?' (critical Parent to Child). The nurse asks 'Is there a social work assessment for Miss Edwards?' (Adult to Adult), to be met by 'Don't ask me, how should I know?' (Child to Parent). The nurse later says 'Please help me make a decision; I'm at my wit's end!' (Child to Parent) to be countered with '**You're** at your wit's end? Just think what it's like for me working with Ethel!' (Child to Parent). All these exchanges are crossed exchanges.

The relationships between the workers would be different had the conversation gone differently:

Nurse: Here is Miss Edwards's medical report. (Adult to Adult)
Social worker: Thank you very much, that will be useful. (Adult to Adult)
Nurse: Is there a social work assessment? (Adult to Adult)
Social worker: Yes, but Jean was meant to bring it and she has been held up. (Adult to Adult)
Nurse: Please help me make a decision; I'm at my wit's end! (Child to Adult)
Social worker: You poor thing. It must be hard. But you are doing all you can. (nurturant Parent to Child)

response from the other person) or crossed (a message from one ego state gets an unexpected response from the other person). Crossed transactions create resentment.

Games

There are a number of classic roles that appear in lots of different scripts and are acted out in what are known as psychological **games**.

Games can be played anywhere. Berne suggests we all play games but are generally unaware that we are doing so. Unknowingly we play our games by seeking others that know the roles and will play opposite roles.

Games tend to be repetitious and predictable and to exploit weakness in one of the people involved. Sometimes we know we are caught up in a pattern of interaction that is always the same and leads nowhere. Nevertheless we play out our parts.

Classic roles (ones that occur in different games) are those of the Victim, Persecutor and Rescuer.

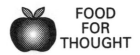

FOOD FOR THOUGHT

Can you identify common phrases attached to the roles of Victim, Persecutor and Rescuer in your workplace?

In your own work settings:

- Who seems to play the victim and in what situations?
- Who seem to play the persecutor and in what situations?
- Are nurses required to be rescuers? In what situations?

In your health care team can you identify any games that are played including Victim, Persecutor and Rescuer?

Two common games that have been identified in nursing situations are 'Yes, but' and 'Kick me'.

'Yes, but': Victim presents a problem; Rescuer gives some advice; Victim switches to Persecutor who then gives 'reasons' why the advice won't work. Rescuer may end up feeling like a Victim after several rounds of this game.

'Kick me': Victim expects to be put down and Persecutor obliges by putting her/him down. Here, Victims may appear to be open and apologetic, but in ways that encourages Persecutors to reprimand them.

There are many other recurring games that people play, but equally there may be some that you come across that are unique to the situations you work in and the people you work with. It is only with insight into the way we and others manage our interactions that we can become more effective in interpersonal skill and avoid playing the kinds of ritualistic games that put ourselves and others down.

SUMMARY

This section has been concerned with the nature of social roles, rules and routines or rituals, taking interaction openings and closures, and transactional analysis as examples. Specifically, the following issues were raised:

- Sequences or episodes of interactions often follow regular patterns.
- These patterns of behaviour are linked to the role–rule context in which they occur.
- Roles are defined by (sets of) expectations.
- Role expectations derive from the (sub)culture, the situation and other people.
- Role conflict or strain occurs as a consequence of different sets of expectations.
- Role conflict or strain usually results in an attempt to reduce/resolve the discomfort.
- Socialization is the means whereby we learn the rules associated with particular roles.
- Social rules or norms derive from the wider social/cultural context or form within groups.
- Social rules or norms underlie patterns or rituals in social behaviour.
- Two examples of highly structured, ritualized routines are interaction openings and closures.
- Openings and closure episodes consist of verbal and non-verbal elements and vary in their length and complexity.
- Social task/cognitive functions can be identified for both openings and closures.
- Social rituals vary with the role–rule context.
- People from similar (sub)cultures share an understanding of important social rituals
- Breakdown in social relations may occur as a result of misunderstanding of social rituals.
- Interpersonal skill does not reside solely in the individual, but is instead a product of the role-rule context.
- Transactional analysis offers another way of misunderstanding rules, roles and rituals.

- We know scripts that are determined by our socialization and roles and organizations we work in.
- Social interaction can be understood as exchanges between Adult, Parent and Child ego states.
- Transactions can be crossed or complementary.
- Psychological games played between people can be identified.

SELF-DEVELOPMENT EXERCISES

1. Think of any three roles you occupy. Where does role conflict come from? Consider the role expectations, demands made by others and pressures due to additional roles you occupy. How do you resolve both role strain and role conflict?
2. With a colleague, discuss what it means to identify with your professional group of nurses. Are there any circumstances in which this identification contributes to thoughts, feelings or behaviours that are either competitive or co-operative with people from other professional groups? What are the circumstances?
3. Describe as fully as you can appropriate interaction openings for the following:
   - As you walk down the ward, you notice a young male patient rearranging his pillow angrily against the back-rest and thumping them noisily as he does so.
   - You are a nurse on a paediatric ward. A mother walks out of a side room, as you are passing, with her young baby in her arms. The baby is supposed to be barrier-nursed. You approach her.
   - The consultant physician is coming to do her ward round. You are in charge of the ward. You want to talk to her about the bed state before she sees her patients.
   - You are making a bereavement visit to an elderly man who has recently lost his wife. The client looks upset when he opens the door to your knock.
4. Describe as fully as you can appropriate interaction closures for the following:
   - You are the theatre nurse who has been undertaking the pre-operative visit to a young female patient who has been scheduled for surgery the following morning. How do you leave the discussion?
   - You have been talking to a distressed relative in a side ward. A colleague rushes in to say your help is needed with a cardiac arrest on the ward. What might you say?
   - You are working in the community. While visiting an elderly woman, you try to convince her of the benefits of losing some weight. She is adamant that she is unable to lose weight, and has

been telling you of her skills as a cook. You have a busy schedule and must leave her. How might you end the visit?

- You have been talking to a junior colleague about some changes that are to be introduced in the service. He is unhappy about his future prospects and wants to talk to you about the possibility of changing jobs. You have to get back to your work. How do you leave the discussion?

5. Talk to some friends or colleagues about different ways of making and accepting apologies. Discuss the different rules for different situations and any cultural differences you have come across.

6. Pay particular attention to a discussion within your work team. What ego-states are being expressed by different people? Note down some crossed transactions that take place. What impact do they have for the progress of the discussion?

7. With a colleague, discuss the concept of interaction games. What games are played regularly in your place of work? What part(s) do you and other people play?

8. Write down a short extract of conversation that has taken place at work. Identify the ego-states that are being expressed, the roles that are being adopted and any games that are being played. How important are the relationships that already exist between people in this situation for the games that are being played? Do the same people play the same roles and games in different situations and with a variety of other people?

CHAPTER 7

Facilitation and the development of rapport

One of the most important things about our interactions with each other is the extent to which we enjoy them. When we come to think just what it is that makes an interaction enjoyable, we can usually point out that it has been rewarding in some way, i.e. we have 'got something out of it'. Generally, we only form relationships with other people on a friendly basis if the rewards of doing so outweigh the costs (Chadwick-Jones, 1976; Gergen, Morse and Gergen, 1980). The more rewards there are, the stronger the relationship will be, and it is reward or satisfaction that keeps the relationship going (Argyle and Henderson, 1985). (It is rather different if we have a role relationship with someone, such as sister–staff nurse, nurse–patient, and so on, as we will find there are often task-related activities associated with the role that force us to interact.)

However, not all the encounters we have in our different roles are connected to tasks. We may simply be chatting to pass the time, keeping each other company, reassuring each other, explaining things to each other or getting to know each other on an informal basis; this is particularly true of many nursing interactions (Cormack, 1985; Hunt, 1991; McLeod Clark, 1983). For these casual encounters, and for those that are related to the emotional needs of one or other of the inter-actors, we know that we need to be able to 'develop a rapport' with our partner. Unless we do this we are likely to find that our relation-ships are unsatisfying, not at all enjoyable and superficial (Knight and Field, 1981; Peterson, 1988). Rewardingness has itself been seen as a social skill (Dickson, Saunders and Stringer, 1993).

RAPPORT

In order to develop a rapport, we must be able to pick up all the cues (verbal and non-verbal) that tell us something about our partners' inner feeling or emotions and their attitudes towards themselves, us and the situation they are in (Mucchielli, 1972). Moreover, we must be able to let our partners know that we have picked up these signals, that we understand them and that as far as possible we will try to meet any needs they have expressed.

Facilitation skills are the ones we use to make interactions rewarding and to develop and maintain rapport. They are not easy skills to use effectively and misunderstandings will often occur. Even if we are quite good at using these skills in some situations, there will be others in which we are not so adept.

In this chapter, we are going to look at some of the issues relating to what we can do to make conversations interesting, how we pick up cues to emotion and interpersonal attitudes and the specific value of self-disclosure.

THE RECOGNITION AND EXPRESSION OF EMOTION

Our ability to develop a rapport depends on whether we can accurately recognize other people's inner feelings or emotional states, whether we can communicate this recognition and whether we can accurately express our own inner feelings appropriately.

The way we recognize others' internal states is to pay careful attention to what they say and, more importantly, what they do. So while people may well say how they are feeling, we often look to the non-verbal cues to get information of how they are **really** feeling (Ekman and Friesan, 1969; Ekman, Friesan and Ancoli, 1980). When we talk about emotion, it is useful to think in terms of the six general emotions and the umpteen other, more specific emotions that are generally considered to be combinations of the six (Trower, Bryant and Argyle, 1978). Table 7.1 gives a rough guide to this way of categorizing emotion.

Different non-verbal cues (or combinations of cues) are associated with different emotions, though we probably rely on the face and the voice for most information.

Other non-verbal cues serve to increase the strength of a feeling expressed. So, for example, tone of voice, body movement, eye contact and gestures can all increase or decrease the intensity of feeling expressed.

Table 7.1 General and specific emotion (from Kagan, Evans and Kay, 1986)

Angry	*Happy*	*Sad*	*Afraid*	*Disgusted*	*Surprised, interested*
Annoyed	Pleased	Sorry	Anxious	Shocked	Amazed
Enraged	Satisfied	Hurt	Alarmed	Sickened	Curious
Irritated	Relieved	Disappointed	Worried	Contemptuous	Fascinated
Frustrated	Thrilled	Regretful	Confused		Intrigued

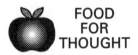

FOOD
FOR
THOUGHT

In what situations do stationary expressions reveal emotional states?

Do some people have fixed facial expressions?

Would the same non-verbal cues to emotions mean the same if displayed by people of a) different ages and b) different cultures?

Does the same expression of emotion mean something different in different situations?

What leads us to make mistakes about how other people are feeling?

Are there any particular cues that 'leak' emotion?

Are there any emotions that a) nurses or b) patients might try to hide? What are they?

What advantages or disadvantages are there in hiding feelings as a) nurses or b) patients?

Are some emotions more easily expressed than others?

Consider, for example, the angry patient who has been sent home after waiting all day for a bed. We know her anger is increasing if she begins waving her arms about, moving closer and raising her voice. Similarly, a patient talking to the stoma nurse reveals increasing despair as she talks more slowly and quietly, looks down more and keeps very still.

Meaning

In Western society, a great deal is made of the need to control our emotions and nursing is, perhaps, one job where there is even more pressure to do so (Llewellyn, 1989). What this really means is that we are expected to control the **expression** of emotion, and it is interesting to note that we are, on the whole, very good at controlling our facial and vocal cues. We still give ourselves away, though, by not paying attention to certain other non-verbal cues that 'leak' contradictory messages.

Consider, for example, the patient, living at home with myeloma. She has generally been well groomed, cheerful and engaging when the community nurse visits. One day, though the nurses notice that she looks unkept and talks very little. The change from her usual way of being may well reveal a mood change. It is very difficult to judge someone's mood on one occasion. By seeing them in different situations and at different times we are able to pick up changes in mood.

When we think we know the 'real' feeling someone is expressing, because we have picked up certain non-verbal cues, despite her/his attempts to control them, there is the danger that we are wrong. We may be picking up cues that do not, in fact, mean anything. The behaviours are habits. This can cause problems when there are wider social interpretations about the emotional meaning of habits. Nail biting and fidgeting with the hands are widely thought, for example, to be signs of anxiety. They may be if people suddenly start to behave in that way. On the other hand, they may not.

So, even if we accurately perceive or notice what is going on, we can only make sense of it if we understand the context in which it occurs. It is the failure to take the context into account that sometimes leads us to make mistakes in judging the inner feelings of others. Context, in this sense, can mean the situation in which the person is or, more generally, their life history. 'I have always bitten my nails' is a statement about context. 'I always bite my nails before job interviews' is a statement about situational context.

The context of emotion

Our understanding of the context is also important if we are to know when and where it is appropriate to express an emotion, and what the acceptable way of expressing that emotion will be.

Display rules

There are rules that tell us when and how to express our feelings, depending on the culture and subcultures to which we belong. These rules are known as 'display rules' (Marsh, Rosser and Harré, 1978; Von Cranach and Harré, 1982; Walsh and Ford, 1989).

Consider for example the child that screams before an injection; the middle-aged patient who weeps when his test results indicate he does not have a malignant tumour; the nurse that cries in the office when a patient dies. All these examples may be considered acceptable. However, small variations might render them unacceptable. So, for an adult to scream before an injection, a middle-aged man to weep when his dinner arrives on time or a nurse to cry on the ward may be inappropriate. In making these judgements we bring our cultural knowledge to bear and our understanding of what is right and wrong in different situations, and in different roles.

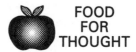

FOOD FOR THOUGHT

Does the recognition of an emotion differ from the interpretation of that emotion? In what ways?

What limits on the expression of different emotions are imposed on nurses?

Are some people more emotional than others? In what ways?

Are we aware of the rules governing the expression of emotion?

What cultural differences are there in Britain in a) the emotion felt and b) the way it is expressed?

Display rules tell us when and how to display emotion. Different rules refer to the events that are 'allowed' to raise particular feelings and the manner in which they should be expressed.

Emblematic behaviour

We also learn that sometimes facial expressions are used to communicate messages that have nothing to do with the expression of emotion, but still have a social meaning. Facial expression, for example, changes when we recognize someone, greet them or depart from them.

Used like this, facial expression is being used 'emblematically', and it is the context again that lets us know when a certain signal is being used to convey a particular feeling, or whether it is being used emblematically. If we confuse the two, we will make a mistake in interpreting what is going on (Nisbett and Ross, 1980).

Labelling emotional states

We use the context, too, to label an inner feeling we have as one emotion rather than the other (Schachter and Singer, 1962). It is the context then that makes us say we are nervous rather than thrilled when we are going to give our first injection, even though we would feel the same sensations when we get the job we really wanted. Thus we label the emotion (and express it differently) according to the context or situation we are in. In other words, our thoughts or cognitions about the situation we are in lead us to label the feelings we have.

We have looked, above, at the cues we use to recognize and express different emotional states, and at those cues that 'leak' information relating to inner feelings. We have considered the importance of the context in its relation to display rules, telling us when and how to express different emotions, and in labelling our own internal states. We will now go on to consider the nature of interpersonal attitudes and their role in interaction.

THE RECOGNITION AND EXPRESSION OF INTERPERSONAL ATTITUDES

Feelings that we have towards other people are called **interpersonal attitudes**, and like emotions, we recognize them by what people do, rather than by what they say. In fact, in the course of our everyday lives we rarely tell someone exactly what we feel towards them, although we may leave them in little doubt (Goffman, 1967).

We can think of our attitudes towards others as reflecting two central attitude dimensions, which are friendly/warm to hostile/cold, and dominant/superior to submissive/inferior (Asch, 1946; Fiske and Taylor, 1991). Thus, we relate to others in terms of liking or affiliation and status. Other common feelings we have are combinations of these two dimensions, and examples are:

- boring;
- pleasing;
- tolerant;
- despairing;

- interesting;
- anxious;
- protective;
- frustrating;
- patronizing;
- relaxing;
- defensive;
- dependent.

Although we use non-verbal information to judge another person's attitude towards us, the timing of a statement may also be a powerful way to communicate an attitude.

No single non-verbal cue relates to a particular attitude. Rather, it is clusters of non-verbal behaviours that we respond to, with different clusters representing affiliative, hostile, dominant and submissive styles. A guide to the usual combinations of cues in the expression of liking and dominance is shown in Table 7.2.

The context of interpersonal attitudes

We do not normally express what we feel when we feel it, but rather decide how and what to communicate, depending on the situation (Goffman, 1967).

As with emotions, there are cultural and subcultural differences in the expression of interpersonal attitudes. What we may think is a friendly approach, for example, may be interpreted as quite insulting, by someone from another culture, and *vice versa*.

Culture and subculture

It is important to realize some of the cultural differences in the communication of interpersonal attitudes, in order to avoid getting hold of the wrong end of the stick and making mistakes.

Consider, for example, the young Pakistani mother who appears diffident and unfriendly. She may be shy, embarrassed and unused to talking to health professionals. Similarly the friendly, chatty youth from the North East of England may be assumed to be unconcerned about his forthcoming CT scan. His behaviour is

Table 7.2 Combinations of cues to liking and dominance (from Kagan, Evans and Kay, 1986)

Focus	Affiliative style	Dominant style
Face	Positive, e.g., interest, smiling	Relaxed, neutral or frowning
Gaze	Long and frequent looks; eye contact	Fewer but longer looks; breaks gaze last
Voice	Soft, low and resonant	Loud, deep tone
Distance	Fairly close (within 1 m)	Either fairly close or fairly distant
Touch	Hand on arm	None
Position	At about 245° angle	Directly in front
Posture	Open arms and either partially open or loosely crossed legs; forwards lean or moderate sideways lean	Reclining angle, relaxed limbs sprawled, shoulders squared, chest expanded
Orientation	Head and shoulders to each other	Either face to face or offset more than 45°
Speech	Listener responses. Speaker disclosures of similarity. Few speech disturbances, good timing. Handing over conversations	Few reflections. Speaks at length. Quick responses and interruptions, asks questions and changes topics. Initiates and closes encounters, expresses different opinions

easily misinterpreted if we do not have good grasp of cultural
norms. The way we interpret the meaning of behaviour can, of
course lead us to miss important clinical signs. Take, for example
the 93-year-old woman living at home with her sister. The community nurse is visiting following her discharge from hospital
after a fall in which she fractured her shoulder. When she gets
there she finds the woman surly, quiet and withdrawn. Coming
away, thinking 'What a miserable old woman she is!' the nurse
misses the possibility that she is depressed. It can be very difficult
for us to appreciate that someone else's behaviour may not mean
what we think it does. We have a tendency to jump to conclu-
sions about the meaning of behaviour.

Roles

Roles often differ from each other in terms of status. We should not be
particularly surprised or upset to find that the ward sister behaves as if
she were superior to her student nurses on the ward, as she has some
legitimate superiority in terms of seniority. If, however, she were to
treat another sister or her nursing officer as inferior, this would be
inappropriate. Similarly, if she met one of her student nurses on
holiday, it would be inappropriate for her to act in a superior manner.

Thus, to make sense of interpersonal attitudes, we need to have an
understanding of the culture/subculture to which people belong, the
role they occupy and the situation they are in, as well as being able
to perceive and interpret different clusters of non-verbal behaviours
(Nisbett and Ross, 1980).

Once we have understood the emotion or interpersonal attitude
being expressed, we must be able to communicate that understanding
if we are to develop a rapport with our partner (Fiedler, 1950). It is the
communication of understanding that we will go on to consider.

THE COMMUNICATION OF UNDERSTANDING

The most common way we communicate understanding is by listening
to what our partner is telling us. When we listen we do not just sit
passively while our partner talks, we actively let her/him know that
s/he is being attended to, heard and understood.

Listening

We use different listening skills on different occasions and for different
purposes, and our behaviour varies along a dimension of activity

(Burnard, 1989). Sometimes it is enough for us to sit quietly still, alert, looking in the general direction of our partner and engaging in direct eye contact; we might use small vocalizations ('Mmm', 'Uh-huh', 'Oh, I see', etc.) and pronounced gestures such as head nods. This is known as **minimal listening**, and we must be careful that we do not slip into minimum attention, go into 'automatic pilot' and cease to really respond.

When we listen to somebody who is obviously emotional, we need to be more active still, and use the skill of reflecting. Basically, reflecting is the ability to let our partner know that we really have heard both the factual and emotional content of what they have said or communicated non-verbally. We have to be careful when we reflect not merely to repeat what the person has said word for word, as to talk to a 'parrot' is at best irritating and at worst insulting and unpleasant. True reflections are difficult to do well, and it is a good idea to practise paraphrasing what people say and finding a few words that sum up quite complicated feelings (Nelson-Jones, 1983).

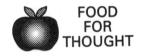

FOOD FOR THOUGHT

What is the difference between attending and listening?
  What role does questioning play in listening?
  How do we know when we are being listened to by someone?
  Is it possible to be over-attentive? What effect does it have?
  What is it like to know we are not being listened to?
  How does listening to someone on the telephone differ from listening to them face-to-face?

In some situations, particularly if someone is finding it difficult to tell us something, we may need to ask questions as part of our listening technique (Epting, 1984). Questions are part of a listening skill when they are used to encourage our partners to continue or elaborate on what they were saying.

At times we may want to offer a personal commentary on what people say, again to encourage them to speak or to think of things connected to what they are saying about which they might otherwise not have thought. As long as the commentary is used to make it easier for our partner to talk further, it is still a listening skill.

Thus we can see that the more active the listening, the more it requires us to speak in focused ways.

Empathy

If we are to be really effective listeners, we must develop the ability to 'take the role of the other', or see things from the other person's point of view. If we are able to do this, we can empathize with that person. Rogers (1975, 1980) argued that empathic understanding is characterized by sensitively and accurately understanding another person's feelings and personal meanings and by communicating this to him or her in a way that does not suggest any attempt at external control (Nelson-Jones, 1983). Rogers does not suggest we have to identify with the other person (and 'become' her or him) but that we should understand what she or he is saying and feeling from her or his own perspective.

It is easy to confuse empathy with sympathy, and indeed we use many of the same techniques in the communication of both empathy and sympathy. Many of the non-verbal behaviours we use to reassure patients, such as close proximity, prolonged eye contact, touch, calm soothing voice, etc. are all part of empathy, but often we will say something as well (Gould, 1990). We have mentioned reflections above, and these can be used to communicate empathy; we can communicate 'advanced empathy' by attempting to draw threads between different conversations, or point to themes that emerge over several occasions and suggest connections that our partners may not have thought of for themselves (Traux and Carkhuff, 1967). This technique is similar to some of those used in social problem solving (see Sections 7.1 and 8.2), but when we use it to convey empathy we are concerned with the emotional content of the conversation. Advanced empathy is particularly important when we are involved with another person over some time in what might be seen as a counselling relationship.

Touch

Touch is a signal that is of great significance for us in nursing (Estabrooks, 1987; Estabrooks and Morse, 1992), both because we use it a lot in just carrying out many nursing tasks, and because if we use it judicially in times of emotional distress it can be a powerful therapeutic and empathic tool (Lorensen, 1983; White, 1988). Despite its obvious use in nursing, Estabrooks and Morse (1992) suggest that relatively little is known about the concept of touch, the development of touching styles or the meaning of touch to nurses, patients or relatives (Jones and Yarbrough, 1985; Nguyen, Heslin and Nguyen, 1975). The importance of understanding the meaning of touch is highlighted by McCain and McKenna (1993). The only touch behaviour perceived as comfortable by the elderly people in their study was instrumental touching of the arm and shoulder by a female nurse.

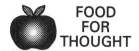

FOOD FOR THOUGHT

Is there a useful distinction to be made between instrumental, caring and protective touch in nursing?

How do nurses learn when and how to touch?

Is touch something that can be learnt or are some people more 'touchy' than others?

How can we begin to understand the meaning of touch in nursing?

What 'rules' are there for nurses touching men and women; old and young patients; people from different cultures? How is knowledge of the rules acquired?

Are there any nursing situations in which touch is difficult? Why is this?

We are often required, for both active listening and empathy, to reveal things about ourselves, i.e. to engage in self-disclosure. Indeed, when and how much to disclose is a very big problem for us as nurses, and when we think about it the issue becomes one of how and if we should keep our role boundaries.

SELF-DISCLOSURE

Self-disclosure refers to the verbal aspects of self-presentation and particularly to information about ourselves that others could not share if we did not reveal it (Jourard, 1964, 1971). Thus self-disclosure differs from self-description, which refers to the information that other people can easily get about us (for example, 'I am a staff nurse', 'I am 30 years old' and so on). We can disclose factual information ('I have been in hospital'), emotions ('I am afraid of anaesthetics'), general feelings ('I like people') or specific feelings ('I like Sister Evans'). Disclosures can be used as part of empathy, and can be varied according to whether they are genuine or apparent. Genuine disclosures are those of a personal nature that we may find embarrassing to reveal, so that when we do it is an indication that we trust the recipient of the information and, since trust is generally thought to be rewarding, this is likely to lead to greater intimacy. We use apparent disclosures in situations where the sharing of information (rather than feeling) is expected. Apparent disclosures are not particularly embarrassing and result in the experience of a pleasant encounter, rather than the development of trust. Since we experience both trust and reciprocity (sharing) as rewarding, both types of disclosures help the development of rapport.

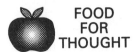

FOOD FOR THOUGHT

Are there cultural differences in the use of self-disclosure?
When does self-disclosure become boasting?
Do people make specific self-disclosures to nurses? Why is this?
What are the disadvantages of self-disclosing, as a nurse?
How can we be sure what is meant when someone self-discloses?

The context of self-disclosure

The use of self-disclosure does not always lead to the development of rapport. If it is not the right time or place to divulge certain information, we may find that the people we are talking to become uncomfortable and end up disliking us (Nelson-Jones and Dryden, 1979; Nelson-Jones and Strong, 1976).

Consider, for example, the patient who insists on telling everyone at the meal table about the pain he feels passing urine. He is likely to cause embarrassment and to be disliked. The health visitor, too, who tells the young mother at home with a difficult baby how she found it difficult to manage with her own son while she was working may find this distances her from the mother. All the mother can see is someone with status (a health visitor), job and obviously coping, whereas she is not. She sees no point of contact between them.

The rules of self-disclosure

To have some idea of the value of making a self-disclosure, we need to know something about the norms or rules underlying situations. This will help us know if self-disclosure is acceptable or not.

There are also rules relating to whether we should reveal positive or negative information about ourselves, even of an impersonal nature (apparent disclosure). Generally we will embarrass people if we reveal intimate information early on in our relationships with them. Trust is needed before this can be done.

There is a belief that nurses should take care to 'protect' themselves and not get too involved with patients, and remain detached. This may be one way we can cope with the extensive emotional demands of the job (Gow, 1982; Llewellyn, 1989). By not using disclosures, we will be better at keeping our distance, but this may be at the expense of not allowing ourselves to develop rapport with patients. This may in turn mean that we are not as helpful to patients as we could be. Rather than ensuring we keep this distance, we might find that we (and patients) experience less distress and more satisfaction if we allow ourselves the freedom to choose when and where to use self-disclosures. Our task will then be one of judging the appropriateness of a disclosure and of striking a balance between the positive effects of conveying empathy and developing rapport and the negative effects of over-involvement.

Of course, self-disclosures are threatening, as there is always the possibility that our 'real' selves will not be liked; and this is especially true of genuine disclosures. We should bear this in mind when patients or colleagues have summoned up the courage to tell us something they think is personally important and we feel the urge to treat it lightly.

SUMMARY

This chapter has been concerned with the skills that are needed to establish and maintain rapport in interaction, that is with facilitation skills. Specifically, the following issues were raised:

- Facilitation skills are used to develop and maintain rapport.
- If rapport is to develop, interactions must be rewarding.
- The accurate recognition and expression of emotions and inter-personal attitudes are central to the establishment of rapport and to ensuring that interaction will be rewarding.
- There is often a discrepancy between the recognition and the inter-pretation of emotions and interpersonal attitudes.
- The change from a person's usual way of behaving is the key to understanding the meaning of her/his behaviour.
- Emotions and interpersonal attitudes can only be fully understood if the social context is taken into account.
- The social context determines the display rules of emotional expression and gives information regarding the norms that dictate how and when to reveal interpersonal attitudes and to use self-disclosure.
- Listening is one of the most important facilitation skills.

- Effective listening varies from less active to more active, i.e., from giving attention by using minimal vocalizations to reflecting the verbal and emotional content of the message to asking questions, to giving a personal commentary.
- The more active the listening, the more likely that empathy is conveyed.
- Empathy includes the willingness to self-disclose.
- Self-disclosures may be of information or feeling, they may be genuine or apparent and they may be positive or negative.
- The social context (including roles and relationships) determines the appropriateness of a disclosure.
- Appropriate disclosures are rewarding and strengthen relationships. Inappropriate disclosures are embarrassing and weaken relationships.

SELF-DEVELOPMENT EXERCISES

1. With a friend, try to describe the combinations of verbal and non-verbal cues that go together to communicate the following emotions: anger, fear, happiness, disgust, sadness, interest, surprise. Do these combinations vary in children and in people from different cultural backgrounds? How does illness affect the expression of emotion?
2. As a nurse, are there any situations in which it would be inappropriate to express any particular emotion? What are they? How do nurses learn these 'display rules'? What happens if the rules are broken?
3. Find some pictures of nurses at work. With a friend, discuss the attitudes towards colleagues, patients or relatives conveyed by the nurses in the pictures. How do you know what these attitudes are? How do misunderstandings in the communication of interpersonal attitudes arise? What different display rules for interpersonal attitudes are there for children and people from other cultural backgrounds?
4. Hold a conversation with a colleague and listen to her/him. Start off by giving her/him your full attention and then move on to minimal listening (with head nods and small utterances) and then more active listening (with summaries of what has been said and so on). Discuss the impact of different types of listening.
5. Discuss with a group of colleagues the difference between empathy and sympathy. Have you ever felt that someone empathized with you? Describe what it was like.
6. Explore different kinds of touch with a friend. One of you should sit in a chair and the other should stand behind and put you hands on her/his shoulders. Discuss how this feels and how it might feel

differently if the person standing was a stranger. Change your touch from 'snowflake' touch to 'raindrop' touch to 'thunderstorm' touch. What different things might be communicated by the different types of touch? Discuss the different meanings the different types of touch might have if applied to different parts of the body.

7. Think of a time when someone talking to you used self-disclosure a) appropriately and b) inappropriately. What impact did each have on you? What made one self-disclosure appropriate and one inappropriate?

8. With a friend, design a nurse training session that is aimed at helping nurses build trust with patients. What key components would you incorporate? How might you prepare nurses for difficulties they might encounter in building trust with: a) male patients; b) female patients; c) children; d) patients who do not speak English?

CHAPTER 8

Influence and assertion

Chapter 7 was concerned with the concept of rewardingness in inter-actions, underlying facilitation skills. This is only one set of skills that can be mustered in response to our goals for a particular interaction. The other skills are those associated with assertion and influence. In this chapter we will examine the place of influence in social interaction generally, and go on to consider, specifically:

- the use of questions;
- the giving of information and explanation;
- assertiveness.

CONTROL AND SOCIAL INTERACTION

Interpersonal relationships may be seen as systems of mutual influence (Durkin, 1988). The way we think about ourselves, the values and the attitudes we hold, the people we associate with, the groups we identify with and our day to day reactions are all due in part to the influence of others. Symbolic interactionist, psychodynamic (including transactional analysis) social learning, humanistic, cognitive and other intergroup perspectives on interpersonal behaviour all stress, in different ways, the effects of others on our behaviour (Bandura 1977, 1986; Berne, 1964; Leyens and Codol, 1988; Rogers, 1980; Stone and Farberman, 1970; Tajfel, 1982b). In even the most casual interactions, 'speakers' control and influence 'listeners' by talking, so that they have to listen, and *vice versa*. Influence may be uneven in more formal situations, due to the different roles that people have. Sometimes situations arise that may require overt – even physical – control. The notion of influence in the context of interpersonal skills, therefore, ranges from subtle influence with little conscious intent to overt and deliberate direction and regu-lation of others. Influence may be exerted on other people's behaviour, their thoughts or their feelings. In other words, our social behaviour (verbal and non-verbal) will affect how others consequently act, think or feel.

Control and influence is exercised by everyone in any social situation to some degree. Nurses control patients by asking them questions, issuing them with instructions, giving or withdrawing explanations or information, persuading them, reassuring them or even by just passing the time of day with them. Patients control nurses, for example, by asking them questions, withholding or volunteering information, complimenting or criticizing them, taking or refusing to take medication. So we can see that nurses and patients influence each other's behaviours, thoughts and feelings in ways that can be positive or negative. Nurses also control colleagues in a variety of ways and for a variety of reasons. By our behaviour (verbal or non-verbal) we can make colleagues behave in different ways and affect how they think and feel about us, themselves, their work and professional competence and other people. Again, this influence can be positive or negative.

We have seen how listening skills, particularly those depending on non-verbal strategies, regulate conversations. Skilled use of verbal strategies as part of more complex listening skills also serve to regulate conversation. Questioning, probing, clarification and elaboration skills can all be used to elicit conversation and to encourage a speaker to explore a range of experiences (Graesser and Black, 1985). They can also be used to mislead a speaker and channel the conversation in an unhelpful direction.

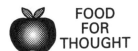

FOOD
FOR
THOUGHT

How easy is it to a) find out information b) encourage talk from someone who is reluctant to say much?

Are different questioning tactics used in different circumstances?

What assumptions underlie the different tactics used (e.g. assumptions about the people, their underlying motivations and feelings, the answers you expect, the situation, etc.)?

How are different questioning tactics used in various nursing situations? How do they vary with age, sex or race of the speakers?

QUESTIONS AND INTERPERSONAL CONTROL

We have seen (Chapter 6) that questions may be used to open conversation and initiate social interaction. They may also be used to elicit personal and medical information, to ascertain attitudes, opinions and feelings, to show interest in a topic or another person, to identify needs, to assess a person's knowledge or understanding, to help con-

Table 8.1 Social functions of questions (from Kagan, Evans and Kay, 1986)

1. To initiate interaction	
Casual, informal openings	N: Hello, you're new, aren't you? P: Have you got a minute, please?
To arouse interest/motivation	N: Who do you think is coming to see you this afternoon? P: Nurse – should the blood be coming up the tube like this?
To show interest and concern	N: Are you all right in there? P: What are you so happy about?
To orientate a task group	N: Is everyone clear what we are doing this afternoon?
2. To obtain information	
Facts	N: Have you had any illness in childhood? N: Do you have someone to bring in your things for you? P: When will the assessment be done? P: What is that drip for?
Attitudes/feelings/opinions	N: How do you feel about going home so soon? N: What do you think about the physiotherapy sessions? P: Would you let your child have the whooping cough jab? P: What do you think about the NHS reforms?
3. To guide conversation	
Change the subject	N: I see, but when did you first feel uncomfortable? P: I understand that lunch is at 12, but when am I going for a scan?
Encourage thought about the future	N: How do you think your husband will cope when you go into hospital? P: Who will do it for me when you are off next week?
Assessment	N: How has your family taken the news? P: Have you changed one of these dressings before?
Clarification	N: What is it you're worried about? P: Do you want me to roll my sleeve right up?
Clarification of jargon	N: When you said you were **confused**, what did you mean? P: You said my mother was in the first priority band; what did you mean?

Manipulation

N: I think we should leave this just now, don't you?
P: You're not up to dealing with people like me are you?

4. To identify problems and needs
Precision

N: When exactly did these anxious feelings start?
P: How long will I have to wait for a decision?

Judge extent of existing knowledge

N: Why do you (think) you take these particular drugs?
P: Did the receptionist tell you why I'm here?

Confront emotion

N: You sound very angry: would you like to tell me why?
P: You look fed up: would you rather talk some other time?

Check understanding

N: So, after what I've just told you, will you just run over the procedure for giving yourself the injection?
P: So am I right in assuming that I can only get this operation if I go into another hospital?

Memory

N: Do you remember how to use the machine?
P: What did I ask you?

5. To expand previous points (probing)
Clarification

N: How exactly does your asthma affect you at work?

Relevance to other issues

N: Does your breathing get worse in smoky rooms?
N: How crucial do you think anxiety is in sparking off an attack?

Extension

N: Is there anything else you can tell me about when your asthma occurs?

Accuracy

N: Did you say your breathing was worse at night?

Consensus

N: You disagree about whether her wheezing is better when it's warm: can you come to some agreement about this?

6. To guide action
Requests

N: Can I take some blood from you now?
P: Please may I make another appointment?

Commands

N: Would you like to go back to your bed now, please?
N: Please will you just roll over so I can do the other side?
P: Would you be so good as to hold the door open?

versations go smoothly, to encourage exploration of experiences and to direct action. Dillon (1990) discusses theoretical and practical issues arising from questioning in a variety of different contexts. A summary of the social functions of questioning is given in Table 8.1 (there may be other functions that different questions serve in different situations that are not included).

These functions are not mutually exclusive and a particular question may serve more than one of them. Also, the same question may serve different functions in different situations, and any particular function may be served by a range of different questions.

?

Consider, for example, a community nurse participating in a care management review meeting. When he asks the home support worker 'Are you OK?' we cannot know the function or the influence of the question unless we know something about the relationship between the two people, the point in the meeting the question is asked and certain background information. If the nurse asks the question as he walks into the room, the question may be in order to initiate interaction. If we know the worker has recently been in hospital the question may be a request for information as well as 'set induction'. If we know the worker and the nurse are to present a minority view to the meeting the question may be a statement of solidarity. If the question is asked after the meeting has identified some care goals to be implemented by the support worker, the question may be to help identify any problems she may be expecting. If the question is asked as the meeting is breaking up, and the nurse knows the support worker is to go back to work with a client who assaulted her yesterday it may be being used to identify a different set of concerns she might have.

We can see, then, that this question could serve any one of several functions. These same functions could have been served by different questions. The question used here was imprecise and open to different interpretations. However, ambiguity in the meaning of the question might also arise from its timing and general context.

Some conversation strategies are part of social routines and ritual and do not, in themselves, mean what they appear to (Goody, 1985). Questions are frequently subject to this ambiguity.

Questions are used for different purposes in different situations, and not all the functions will always be relevant. The reasons for using questions at home or in informal settings will be different from at work. The way in which a question is asked in part determines how well it serves the function that was intended. There are different types of question that lead to different types of reply and that are more or less useful. Much of the research (Macleod-Clark, 1983, 1984; Maguire, 1985) into the verbal behaviour of nurses indicates that nurses tend to use inappropriate styles of questioning that result in failures of communication from both their own and patients' point of view. Patients are not given opportunities to explore their feelings, while nurses fail to detect underlying needs and frequently miss the opportunity to gather vital information. Table 8.2 summarizes helpful and unhelpful types of question.

Different situations, coupled with the purpose of questioning, determine which style is most appropriate (Dillon, 1990).

A useful distinction to make is that between **open** and **closed** questions (Burnard, 1989; French, 1983; Long, Paradise and Long, 1981).

Closed questions are the ones that limit the possibilities of reply. They are used in the collection of facts and to discover preferences between given alternatives: frequently they invite yes/no answers and thus do not encourage much talk. The questioner requires prior knowledge about the topic of conversation in order to decide on the most useful question(s) to ask. Because of this, though, valuable information may be lost if s/he has limited knowledge or considers some topics to be unimportant or insignificant. Furthermore, ill-informed use of closed questions can glean information that is irrelevant.

Open questions, on the other hand, allow the respondent the freedom to reply in any way s/he wishes. They encourage talk, as yes/no answers are difficult to make. Because the onus is on the respondent to provide detail, little prior knowledge of the topic is required of the questioner. This means, though, that if the respondent considers information to be unimportant or insignificant it may well be lost. As the content of the reply is unpredictable, the questioner needs considerable skill in taking up cues in order to pursue the conversation meaningfully and to avoid becoming sidetracked. Open questions are particularly valuable in eliciting attitudes, values, opinions and feelings and, as such, may be threatening to either party.

Both closed and open questions can be useful in nurse–patient interaction. There is, as we have said, a tendency to use closed questions when open ones would have been more appropriate. Closed questions undoubtedly give the questioner control over both the conversation and her/his emotional involvement (Pepler and Lynch, 1991).

There are other types of question that are commonly used. They control and determine the course of the interaction and leave people with thoughts and feelings about the questioner that are generally

Table 8.2 Types of question or styles of questioning

Helpful styles: Used appropriately, fulfil many social functions	
Closed questions	
Limit the possibilities of reply	Do you want rice pudding or fruit?
Useful in eliciting facts	How old are you?
	Did you fall on your arm?
Questioner needs prior knowledge	Are you still at this address?
	Is your daughter visiting tonight?
Discourages talk	Does it hurt a lot?
Non-threatening (usually)	Shall I contact your mother?
	Did you go shopping today?
Open questions	
Provide the freedom to answer in any way	How do you feel?
	What happened to you?
Useful in eliciting attitudes, values, feelings, opinions	In what ways does she irritate you?
	How do you feel about your neighbours?
	What do you think about the operation?
Little prior knowledge required	What is the test for?
	What are you in for?
	What goes on here?
Encourages talk	What is it you're worried about?
	What's been happening over the weekend?
	Why do you ask that?
May be threatening	Who should I contact to let them know you're here?

Unhelpful styles: Create ambiguity and confusion

Leading questions

Wording suggests answer — I expect you're looking forward to your holiday, aren't you?

Do you think nurses do a good job?

Statement and/or value contained in question — Shall we go to the canteen now?

Would you like to get the treatment over first?

Encourages the acceptance of premises in subtle ways

May invite respondent to bias answer to reflect (assumed) normative values — You can't wait to get home, can you?

Are you glad your son has offered to help you?

Misleading replies may be given as a result — Are you feeling better now that Doctor's visited you?

Do you understand it now?

Double-barrelled/multifaceted questions

Two or more questions asked as one — Would you like a bath now or shall we have a cup of tea?

Respondent may want to reply to all/some/none of the alternatives — Has the pain gone and the flashes settled down or has it spread to your leg?

Rhetorical questions

Statements posed as questions: no answer generally required — Shall we look at your dressing?

Questioner may go on to provide the answer — Would you like a bath? Let's get you undressed.

Respondent may (mistakenly) provide an answer — You have your test today, haven't you? – I don't think so.

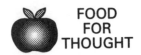

**FOOD
FOR
THOUGHT**

How easy it is to distinguish between open and closed questions?

In what nursing situations are closed questions best used and in what nursing situations are open questions best used?

Are open or closed questions more common in nursing situations? Why might this be?

What consequences do open questions have for a) the questioner and b) the respondent?

What other interpersonal skills are required if a) open and b) closed questions are to be used effectively?

Do a) women and men b) children and adults c) people from different cultural groups differ in their use of open and closed questions? In what ways?

Can you identify the types of question used in this box? How else might these questions have been asked?

unintended. Sometimes, however, the effects they have are intended, in which case they are manipulative. **Leading questions** are those whose wording suggests the answer that is expected. Most leading questions invite the respondent to agree with a statement of fact or value contained within the question.

Consider, for example, the effects that different types of question might have. Leading questions can be subtle and encourage the acceptance of certain premises. This may be what is intended, or it may limit the possible replies, in which case the questioner may be none the wiser after hearing the answer.

The nurse who asks Karen, the suicidal patient, 'There's a lot worth living for, isn't there?' may be trying to get her to find something worth living for. If Karen answers 'Yes', the nurse doesn't know what she means. She may mean 'Yes, if you say so' or 'Yes, but not for me' or 'You haven't listened to a word I've been saying, have you?'. The way Karen answers and what she goes on to say – if anything – will help the nurse decide what effect her question had. She might have asked her question differently, which would have led the conversation in different directions. For instance, she could have asked 'What do you think is worth living for?' or 'Why do you think most people think it's worth carrying on living?' or 'Is there anything you think it's worth living for?' or 'What do you enjoy?', etc. These are all different ways of asking the same thing – assuming that what she was trying to find out was what Karen might feel was (perhaps) worth living for.

All these questions are loaded in one direction and express the assumptions that there is something worth living for or to be enjoyed. It will be the way particular answers are framed that will help the nurse decide how to take the conversation on – but she will have to be skilled in observation and interpretation to pick up sensitively on the replies.

Biases may also be introduced into questions that imply a person should reply in particular ways (because to reply honestly may reveal a personal deviance from some social standard of 'correctness'). Misleading pictures of parents' abilities to handle their adult son with severe learning difficulties may derive from questions such as 'How is he at mealtimes?', 'Is he dry at night', 'How much noise does he make?', 'Are there any problems with bathing him?'

Questions that may leave people confused and elicit misleading replies are those that in effect ask several things at once. Sometimes they may be double-barrelled or multifaceted. The respondent may want to reply to some or all or none of the alternatives.

The final type of question that is often ambiguous, and thereby confusing, is the **rhetorical question**. Rhetorical questions are questions that are really statements and do not require an answer. They are used in conversation as opening and closing gambits, and sometimes defensively in the course of the conversation, with the questioner subsequently providing the answer. The trouble is that sometimes people reply to them.

We have seen, then, that questions are not simply requests for information. They serve many different functions and the skilled choice of style of questioning can ensure that nurses get all they can from interviews with patients, relatives and colleagues. The context or situation will determine what it is that nurses hope to get out of their conversations, and their goals should determine their choice of questioning style. Dillon (1990, p. 145) sums up his discussion of types of questions and the ways they are put by stating 'there is no one form of question and no one manner of asking questions that is reliably known to have one given effect even in given situations'. He goes on to suggest that practitioners are the best people to know how effective their questioning strategy has been in a particular circumstance, The skilled practitioner attends as much – if not more – to answers and answering as to questions and questioning. It is only by listening to the answers that nurses can judge the impact of their questioning and when and how to continue the conversation.

Just as nurses can control interactions through the skilled use of questions, so too can patients. Calls for explanation, information and (sometimes) reassurance are often made, and nurses have to respond to them. The answers they give vary considerably in their skill and thereby their efficacy. Information and explanations are often sought.

REASSURANCE, INFORMATION AND EXPLANATION

Nurses often respond to requests for information with attempts to reassure patients, especially if the information asked for is potentially upsetting for either nurses or patients. Nurses often respond to such situations by avoiding or blocking further discussion of the topic (Menzies, 1960; Macleod Clark, 1984; Kagan, 1979; Wright, 1991). It is sometimes appropriate to give reassurance. However, it will only be effective if nurses first establish what the patient is concerned about and why. If reassurance is used by the nurses as a means of avoiding underlying concerns, it may do little to help the patient.

More commonly, a request that at first appears to be for reassurance is really one for explanation or information. Patients often ask for information about medical/hospital activities and procedure, the nature of their disease, treatment and prognosis, as well as the reasons for their current feelings. The need to give information stems also from nurses. Nurses may want to explain procedures and possible outcomes in order to prepare patients, say, for tests or surgery; they may want to gain patients' co-operation with nursing tasks or to teach them how to undertake the tasks themselves, or they may be responsible for notifying patients of test results and their implications. Patients gain emotionally and physically from being given open and honest information (Davis, 1985; Knight and Field, 1981; Wilson Barnett, 1981). It can be seen, then, that the need for information may stem from patients or nurses or both, and it is necessary to be clear about the origin of the need in order to plan and present the information to its best effect (Hargie, Saunders and Dickson, 1981).

Figure 8.1 outlines the process of giving effective information as suggested by French (1983).

We often fall into the trap of giving explanations prematurely and

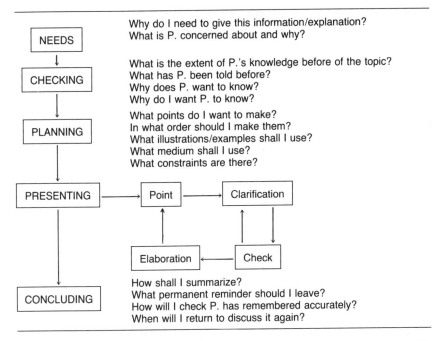

Figure 8.1 The process of giving information–from nurse (N) to patient (P) (from Kagan, Evans and Kay, 1986).

providing too much information at once. It is necessary, therefore, to check the extent of the recipient's knowledge in order to plan what to say and how. At the planning stage, several questions need to be asked. First, will the explanation be written, spoken, recorded or 'live'? Of course some situations require immediate verbal response to a request, in which case this choice may not exist: others, though, permit planning in advance. Second, what are the essential points to be covered and in what order? If the order of importance of points is not carefully considered, then problems of misunderstanding may arise as issues relating to diagnosis, treatment, side effects and prognosis become intermingled. Third, what illustrations or examples will be used to make the explanation more clear and/or memorable? Fourth, what constraints (such as hospital regulations, Sister's instructions, doctors' rules, etc.) dictate what can or cannot be said?

Whether information is prepared in advance or is offered spontaneously, there are several things to be borne in mind in presenting it. Figure 8.2 shows the steps involved in effective information giving.

The final stage of the process is that of concluding. This may involve summarizing what has been said; further checking for understanding; establishing the need, and, if relevant, the time and place for a follow-

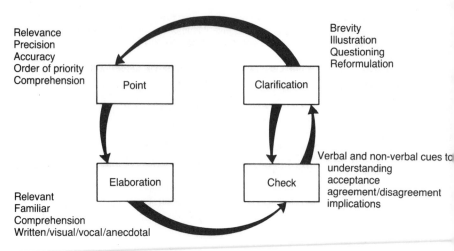

Relevance
Precision
Accuracy
Order of priority
Comprehension

Point

Clarification

Brevity
Illustration
Questioning
Reformulation

Elaboration

Check

Relevant
Familiar
Comprehension
Written/visual/vocal/anecdotal

Verbal and non-verbal cues to
understanding
acceptance
agreement/disagreement
implications

Figure 8.2   Presentation of information (from Kagan, Evans and Kay, 1986).

up session; and leaving a permanent reminder of the major points that had been made.

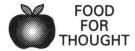 **FOOD
FOR
THOUGHT**

How do you assess the need for giving and receiving information? In what ways does this vary in different situations?

What difficulties might there be in checking understanding prior to giving information and in planning the presentation?

What modifications need to be made when giving information to young and old patients?

In what ways might you help someone remember simple information s/he has been told?

What barriers are there to effective information giving in different nursing settings?

There are some common faults in giving information that occur in different nursing situations. In order to avoid or overcome these faults, it is necessary to notice them occurring and to practise alternative strategies. Sometimes these faults are linked to our personal styles of behaving. The most common are:

- lack of structure resulting in needless repetition;
- use of technical language or jargon contributing to misunderstanding or ambiguity;
- inappropriate style of speech forming a restricted code;
- poor illustrations and examples leading to confusion;
- inaccurate detail resulting from insufficient preparation;
- distortion of the truth and lack of clarity leading to confusion and assumptions;
- inadequate checking what has been understood and remembered resulting in raised anxieties and reluctance to discuss the matter in the future.

From this list we can see that poor information leads to confusion, ignorance and deceit. As such it is often controlling and manipulative (Lanceley, 1985; Ward, 1988). The skilful use of questions and of giving information are effective ways of influencing others and of moving towards clear and honest communications. A further set of skills we can use in pursuit of social goals are those of assertiveness.

ASSERTIVENESS

Assertiveness is a particular form of control, and interest in it as a specific skill has grown in recent years. It is often thought that assertion is the skill of standing up for yourself and getting exactly what you want, either directly or by manipulating other people. Inherent in this notion is the exercise of power over other people. Assertion is not about power: it is better described as the art of confident, clear, honest and direct communication, while at all times retaining respect for other people (Dainow and Bailey, 1988; Dickson, 1982). Assertiveness is non-aggressive, non-defensive and non-manipulative and it does not interfere with other people's freedom to take an assertive stance or make appropriate decisions. To be assertive is not always to get your own way. It may well be that we reach a compromise on all/any of the issue(s). In reaching this position, though, by being assertive we should never compromise our own self-worth (Lindenfield, 1986). All those involved should continue to feel acknowledged and not 'put down' or humiliated. If they do not feel acknowledged, it is likely that the encounter will have been handled aggressively or manipulatively, rather than assertively. (Porritt, 1990; Vaughan and Pillmoor, 1989).

If assertion is not about getting our own way, what is it about? What are known as **assertive rights** are listed below: as Rakos (1991, p. 26) points out 'the expression of rights is the core of any assertion, its *raison d'être*; it is necessary but not sufficient to maximize long-term as well as short-term positive consequences.'

Assertive rights (from Kagan, Evans and Kay, 1986, adapted from Smith, 1975)

Assertiveness is seen to be the articulation of basic rights we have as people, and these are summarized below:

- You have the right to state your own needs and set your own priorities as a person independent of any roles that you assume in your life.
- You have the right to offer no reasons or excuses for justifying your behaviour.
- You have the right to decline responsibility for other people's problems.
- You have the right to change your mind.
- You have the right to make mistakes.
- You have the right to say 'I don't know'.
- You have the right to deal with others without being dependent on them for approval.
- You have the right to be illogical in making decisions.
- You have the right to say 'I don't understand'.
- You have the right to ask for what you want.
- You have the right to say 'Yes' or 'No' for yourself.
- You have the right to express your feelings.
- You have the right to express your opinions and values.
- You have the right to be treated with respect as an intelligent, capable and equal human being.

Are there any 'rights' you would like to add? If so, write them in.

-
-
-
- **You have the right to say 'No' without feeling guilty.**

These are, then, the basic rights we have as people, and assertion is the articulation of these rights. There may be some other 'rights' that we have not included, and space has been left in the list for those to be added.

A criticism that is often raised of this list is that to articulate all these rights would lead to selfishness and a lack of consideration for others. The important things to remember are the following.

- One person's rights are never at the expense of another's. Everyone must be respected at all times.
- What a person does should always be based on her/his assessment of what s/he want to do, and s/he should not be prevented from making such an appraisal. What s/he actually does is her/his own decision, and as such should not be judged by others.
- Along with 'rights' go 'responsibilities' (Lange and Jakubowski, 1978). We should try to clarify the responsibilities that go along with assertive rights.

Most of us experience some difficulty in handling those interpersonal situations that require us to assert ourselves in some way.

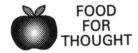

FOOD FOR THOUGHT

How comfortable are you with the concept of 'rights'? Why do you think that is?

Are you generally passive, manipulative, aggressive or assertive? Why?

Does your usual pattern of response vary between work and home? What is the difference and why do you think this is?

How easy do other people make it for you to be assertive? What can you do about this?

Are women more assertive than men? Why?

What is the link between assertiveness and power?

Are there any nursing situations where you do not think it appropriate to be assertive? What are they?

Some basic assertive techniques

There are three components to the skill of assertion, and these are:

- to be able to decide what it is you want or feel, and say so specifically and directly;
- to stick to your statement, repeating it, if necessary, over and over again;

- to deflect assertively any responses from the other person which might undermine your assertive stance.

Vaughan and Pillmoor (1989) suggest some verbal and non-verbal tactics for achieving assertiveness. Verbal tactics include:

- **use 'I' statements**: these help us assume responsibility for our own behaviour and lessen the likelihood that we blame others for what we do (for example, 'I feel annoyed when you leave all the laundry for me' instead of 'You make me annoyed when you don't do the laundry');
- **change verbs** – 'can't' to 'won't' and 'have to' to 'choose to': this helps us see that we have choices and can change our own circumstances if we want to (for example, 'I won't speak up on ward rounds' instead of 'I can't speak up on ward rounds'; 'I choose to work a double shift to cover for a colleague's sick leave' instead of 'I have to work a double shift . . .');
- **self-disclosure**: say what we feel in order to help us relax and begin to take charge of ourselves (for example 'I feel frustrated just now' rather than getting increasingly agitated as a result of rising frustration, possibly culminating in an outburst).

Non-verbal tactics include:

- **voice and speech pattern**: a steady, medium volume, warm voice, accompanied by deep breaths in a difficult situation, helps us be more relaxed and able to be heard clearly;
- **calm facial expression**, relaxed eye contact and relaxed mouth and jaw all help us to convey sincerity and be taken seriously.

Handling feedback

Once we have acquired the basic skills of assertion, we can begin to think of applying them to familiar situations. Receiving feedback, particularly critical feedback, often leaves us feeling angry, hard done by, humiliated or embarrassed and yet critical feedback can be valuable if it is constructive and valid (Vaughan and Pillmoor, 1989). The trouble is, criticism often contains put-downs or unwarranted attacks on us as people. Nevertheless, criticism can be useful and assertiveness includes the ability to ask for, and be open to, constructive criticism as well as a willingness to compromise and change (Lindenfield, 1986). Some aspects of criticisms may well be justified, but some may be unjustified, implying all sorts of hidden meanings. The assertive way to deal with criticism is to confront both these aspects: to acknowledge those parts are justified and to challenge those that are not.

Consider, for example, the outpatient clinic nursing auxiliary who has forgotten to give a patient a form for monitoring the waiting times in clinic.

Clinic sister: All this going off on courses makes you forget what you're doing here.
Auxiliary: I'm sorry I forgot to give her the form (*justified criticism*). I'll note down her times myself (*compromise*). I'll try to make sure I remember to do the rest (*change*).

This reaction to the criticism shows a willingness to accept those parts of the criticism that were valid, a willingness to compromise and to change. This is a very different reaction from one that is defensive and possibly angry, as in the following response to the same situation:

Clinic sister: All this going off on courses makes you forget what you're doing here.
Auxiliary: I don't usually forget, not like some people (*defensive*). These forms are stupid anyway – no-one does anything with them; one missing won't make any difference (*unwillingness to compromise*). I'm jolly well going to go on as many courses as I can and you can't stop me (*beginning to get angry*).

Another way to respond assertively to criticism is to challenge the right–wrong judgements by the critic or to ask for explanation or expansion of the invalid parts of the criticism. These ploys give the critic the chance to be more constructive in her criticism and thus be more assertive herself. Taking the same example again:

Clinic sister: All this going on courses makes you forget what you are doing here.
Auxiliary: I'm sorry I forgot to give her the form (*justified criticism*). What other things do I forget (*request for expansion*)?
or
I have been on a lot of courses recently (*justified criticism*). What problems does this create (*challenge of the right–wrong assumption*)?
or
I'm sorry I forgot to give her the form (*justified criticism*). And I have been on a lot of courses recently (*justified criticism*). How

do you think I could make the most of them in my work (*request for clarification and expansion*)? I would appreciate your help in implementing clinic procedures (*specific request*).

Handling compliments

Interestingly, giving and receiving positive feedback or compliments assertively is often more difficult than dealing with criticism. Compliments, too, generally contain a component that is justified and an arbitrary value judgement, although in this case the value is usually positive. Compliments may be handled in much the same way as criticisms are.

We do have a tendency to deny compliments, to react as though the person offering the compliment was being sarcastic or even rude. In other words we assume a latent meaning to what was said (see Chapter 3). However, if we are to assume that everyone should be enabled to act assertively, then, given the definition of assertion as honest and direct communication, we must take compliments at their face value, not in terms of their latent meaning.

Having said this, though, we are generally well used to using compliments as a means of being sarcastic. On the whole people find it as hard to give genuine compliments as to receive them. For some reason we find the expression of positive feeling towards others as difficult as the expression of negative ones, if not more difficult.

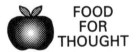 FOOD
FOR
THOUGHT

Are criticisms and compliments more difficult to deal with in some relationships (e.g., between colleagues, doctors and nurses, nurses and patients, peers, friends, relatives, etc.) than others? In what ways?

How does your role affect your ability to handle criticism or compliments?

How are criticism and compliments influenced by age, sex, cultural background?

What tendencies do you have to give or receive criticism or compliments in particular ways? What will it take for you to become more assertive in giving and receiving criticism and compliments?

We have discussed above some of the most common sources of difficulty with assertion, namely handling criticism and giving and receiving compliments.

NEGOTIATION AND COMPROMISE

Assertiveness often requires some negotiation in order to reach a compromise that is acceptable to both (or all) parties. Nurses have to negotiate informally and formally with colleagues, other professionals, patients and relatives in many different situations. Negotiation itself, as well as more general assertive behaviour, requires us to compromise (Fisher and Ury, 1981). There are many different kinds of compromise, but perhaps the most useful distinction is between **retrograde** and **progressive** compromises. Retrograde compromises make matters worse for one of the parties concerned or a third party who will be affected by the decision reached. Progressive compromises, while not

Consider, for example, the community psychiatric nurse who is helping to support Rose, an 87-year-old woman with dementia, in her own home. Rose's niece wants her in a nursing home. The care manager's assessment has put her in the first priority category, eligible for residential care. The nurse thinks she should be helped to stay in her own home. In his view, a place in a nursing home would make matters worse for her (be a retrograde compromise); living with her niece would also make matters worse; frequent short periods in the nursing home would not make matters worse but would not improve things either; increasing home support and help to go to a day centre would not only prevent deterioration but would make more opportunities for social contact; increasing home support and time at the day centre combined with moving the gas fire out of her reach would in addition decrease her risk of burning or setting the room on fire.

There may be many more options, all of which will vary on the retrograde–progressive continuum. To be assertive the nurse will be willing only to consider these which are not retrograde – but this after full exploration of all the issues.

either party's ideal solution, either make things better or maintain the status quo and prevent deterioration for either party involved or any third party affected by the decision. In any discussion or decision that has to be made, there are always different solutions or compromises that can be reached, all of which vary in the extent to which they are progressive or retrograde. Assertiveness requires exploration of these alternatives with the responsibility to ensure the most progressive compromise possible is achieved (Drucker, 1980). Non-assertiveness may either involve manipulation or aggression in order to get our own way, or passivity in giving in and letting others get their own way.

There are other, perhaps more complex assertive skills that nurses require in order to exercise control in their interpersonal lives. The next chapter will discuss the handling of conflict, aggression and violence.

SUMMARY

This chapter has been concerned with basic skills of control in personal encounters, namely the use of questions, giving information and explanation and assertiveness. Specifically, the following issues were raised.

- Control is central to all interpersonal relationships and ranges from subtle influence to deliberate regulation of others.
- Questioning, instructing, explaining and reassuring are frequent forms of control for nurses.
- Questioning serves to elicit information and to encourage a person to explore a range of experiences.
- Questions serve many different social functions in different situations.
- Questions, as part of social rituals, may be ambiguous.
- Appropriate style of questioning is determined by the situation and the questioner's goals.
- Depending on the situation, open and closed questions might be helpful.
- Leading, multiple and rhetorical questions are rarely helpful.
- Information and reassurance are often confused.
- Patients' needs should be assessed prior to giving information/ explanation.
- Giving information involves stages of establishing needs, checking, planning, presenting and concluding.
- The presentation of information requires decisions to be made regarding the issue(s), elaboration(s), levels of understanding and clarification.
- Insufficient attention to how information is given may lead to inaccuracy.

- Assertiveness is the art of confident, clear, honest and direct communication while retaining respect for other people.
- Assertion can be distinguished from passivity, aggression and manipulation.
- Assertion frequently involves reaching a compromise.
- 'Assertive rights' underlie the need to develop skills of assertion.
- Basic assertive techniques include being specific, sticking to the point and deflecting attempts at sidetracking.
- Handling criticism and giving/receiving compliments are sources of difficulty for many people.
- Assertiveness requires negotiation and compromise.
- Compromises can be progressive or retrograde.

SELF-DEVELOPMENT EXERCISES

1. Listen to an interview on the radio or television. What kinds of question does the interviewer use and what kinds of response does s/he get? Write down examples of closed, open, leading, rhetorical and multiple questions.
2. During a patient assessment, identify different types of question that are used. What kinds of question reveal what types of information?
3. With a friend, devise appropriate written or verbal information for patients or relatives in the following situations:
   - precautions to be taken when a family member has food poisoning;
   - medication advice on discharge;
   - catheterizing a patient;
   - monitoring an asthmatic child's response to inhaled medication;
   - collecting a midstream specimen of urine.
   Which stages of the information-giving process are likely to be the most problematic?
4. Rewrite the following passages so they are free from jargon and technical language.
   - Your husband has had a perforated gangrenous appendix that burst. Consequently he's very dehydrated and pyrexial, that's why he's on an IV. There's a tube to drain the gunge from his abdomen. He might look a bit distended but don't worry – this is normal. We will record his vital signs every half hour.
   - Because you have already had one CVA, and as a prophylactic measure to improve your cerebral blood flow, what they will do is to scrape out the inside of the artery going to your brain and widen it. You'll have a GA so you won't feel a thing.
5. Identify the deficiencies in the following information-giving session.
   Staff nurse (talking to newly admitted male patient): 'We think you have had an MI (that's a coronary), so we'll pop you on the cardiac

monitor to record your ECG. I'll just do your BP then Doctor will come and take some blood (only a few mls) from your arm for enzymes. Don't take the leads off, will you, and don't get out of bed. We'll give you something for the pain because it's important that you relax. Don't worry, we'll be monitoring you from the central console to watch for any arrhythmias so you'll be OK. You'll be all right now, honestly!'

6. Watch a television sitcom or soap opera. Try to identify when any character is being a) aggressive, b) manipulative and c) assertive. What do they do or say in each situation, and what impact does it have on other people round them? What are the advantages of being aggressive, manipulative or assertive in different situations?

7. Try to devise assertive replies to the following.
   - Perhaps you had better concentrate properly on one area before you start on another.
   - You know that the quality information forms need to be in the office by 12.10 on Friday. Yours are always late.
   - I'd appreciate it if you'd show some respect. I've got a son older than you.
   - You're all the same, you nurses – what kind of people do they employ nowadays?
   - Your uniform skirt is a bit short, isn't it?

8. Are criticisms and compliments more difficult to deal with assertively in particular relationships? In what ways? How can criticisms be made to be constructive? Are compliments or criticisms easier to give or receive at home or at work? Why?

CHAPTER 9

Counselling

Counselling may be seen as a process whereby one person helps another to clarify her/his life situation and to decide upon future lines of action (Burnard, 1989). Counselling helps people constructively to resolve personal problem(s) that may be long-standing or acute. As Burnard (1989) says: 'The aim of counselling must be to free the person being counselled to live more fully and such fuller living comes through **action** . . . [counselling] . . . must seek to enable the client to become confident enough to choose a particular course of action and see it through' (p. 2).

THE COUNSELLING APPROACH

There are times when the most helpful thing a nurse can do for someone who has a problem is to provide the sort of conditions that will encourage that person to explore the problem and arrive at viable solutions her/himself. In such situations persuasion is no good, re-assurance is difficult and advice giving is inappropriate.

If people are encouraged to recognize their emotional difficulties and find a solution to them, the approach to helping may be called a counselling approach. A useful distinction can be made between nurses-as-counsellors and nurses-using-counselling-skills. Macleod Clark, Hopper and Jesson (1991) suggest that communication skills form the foundation of counselling skills which in turn underpin the process of counselling. Nurses can move from communication to using counselling skills, to counselling with increased self-awareness and specialist skills training.

There are many different kinds of situation in which nurses might effectively use counselling skills or the counselling process. For example, they might be working with patients and their relatives who are undergoing life-threatening illnesses or procedures (Thompson, Webster and Meddis, 1990; Wilkinson, 1991), bereavement or loss (Murgatroyd and Woolfe, 1982), physical impairment of a child (Booth, 1978; Challela, 1981) or patients or colleagues following a traumatic

Consider, for example, the middle-aged man who has an aortic aneurism. He is worried that the pain he has is not controlled adequately. There are a number of different ways the nurse can respond to him when he talks about not being able to concentrate on anything because of the pain. She can **reassure** him the pain will get less and that most people adapt to it reasonably well; she can try to **persuade** him to cope with it without analgesia; she can **sympathize** with him, by saying how awful it must be; she can **advise** him on how to cope with the pain when it is at its worst. None of these responses from the nurse involve the patient in actively exploring his difficulty coping with the pain and the consequences it has for him: nor do they help him identify ways of resolving his difficulty. It may well be that the patient is really more concerned about not being able to read anything, rather than about the pain *per se*; or he may be worried he will die. A **counselling** response may help him clarify what the essential part of his concern is and find personal solutions.

accident (Bowles, 1991; Errington, 1989; Gowins-Rubin, 1990). Broadly, then, the main objectives of nurses as counsellors are:

- to create an atmosphere in which others feel accepted, understood and valued, so that they are helped to explore their thoughts, feelings and behaviour;
- to help others reach clearer understanding;
- to help others find their own strengths to cope more effectively with their lives by making appropriate decisions;
- to support and encourage alternative ways to act;
- to help others evaluate the consequences of their actions, and to plan and engage in further actions if necessary.

This approach is what can be called an eclectic person-centred approach to counselling (Egan, 1986; Carkhuff, 1983). It is based on the work of Rogers (1951, 1957, 1961, 1983). Rogers introduced the idea that three core conditions of empathy, unconditional acceptance and genuineness are essential to the counselling relationship and counselling process. It is only if these conditions are met that people will be able to grow in awareness and resourcefulness. It is important to clarify this, so that we do not become confused with other approaches to counselling (Burnard, 1989; Stewart, 1983). Within this framework, two features distinguish counselling from other forms of helping. Firstly, if nurses are counselling, they are encouraging others to explore and understand their thoughts and feelings, and to work out what they might do before taking action. Secondly the role of the nurse is to help others form decisions or find solutions of their own. Counselling is not a better form of helping, it is a different one and is only the preferred form in some situations.

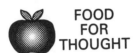

FOOD FOR THOUGHT

What place does counselling have in nursing?

Can counselling take place as part of different helping relationships?

Are some people naturally good at counselling?

How easy is it to be empathic, unconditionally accepting and genuine?

In what circumstances is it difficult for nurses to meet Rogers' core conditions of counselling?

What difficulties arise for nurses counselling work colleagues?

What barriers are there to effective counselling in nursing?

Are there any specific issues arising from using counselling skills with people older or younger, same- or opposite-sex people and people from different cultures?

Very often the transitory and emotionally charged nature of nurses' relationships with others, particularly patients, means that counselling relationships extending over a period of time may be difficult to achieve. However, nurses may still be able to use some of the skills of counselling in order to enrich therapeutic personal relationships (Stewart, 1975).

THE COUNSELLING PROCESS

We have talked above of the counselling relationship and of counselling skills. It is the relationship that creates the helpful atmosphere in which the skills will be used to best effect, and in turn certain skills help create the helping relationship. So, for example, nurses who hope to be able to help others cope with their anxieties about forthcoming surgery will only be able to do so if they have skilfully developed a climate of warmth and trust. Counselling, then, includes skills of building relationships and of helping: one cannot occur without the other (Kennedy, 1977).

A useful way to think about the skills involved in counselling is to

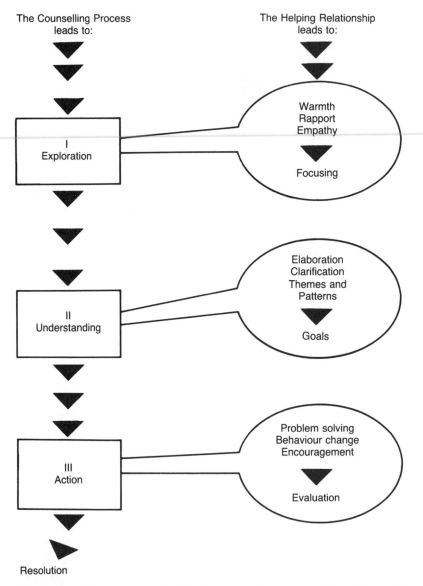

Figure 9.1 Three-stage model of the counselling process (from Kagan, Evans and Kay, 1986).

look at different stages of the counselling process. A three-stage model of counselling is shown in Figure 9.1.

Here, the counselling process leads the client to explore, understand and act, while the helping relationship seeks to establish warmth and rapport, to help clarify problem(s), to set goals and to realize certain courses of action and to evaluate their effectiveness.

Each stage requires counsellors to use specific sets of skills, with later stage(s) building on the skills of earlier stages, as shown below.

Counselling skills for each stage of the counselling process (from Kagan, Evans and Kay, 1986)

Stage I: Exploration
- Attention giving
- Passive listening
- Active listening – communicating empathy, acceptance, genuineness by:
  - paraphrasing
  - reflecting thoughts and feelings
  - summarizing
- Focusing: helping client to be specific
- Moving conversations on

Stage II: Understanding
- All the skills of stage I
- Helping the other to clarify and elaborate
- Offering new perspectives or alternative frameworks
- Listening for themes, patterns or gaps and helping the other to recognize them
- Comforting
- Self-disclosure
- Immediacy: what is happening between counsellor and the other, now
- Timing
- Goal-setting

Stage III: Action
- All the skills of Stages I and II
- Identifying strengths
- Stimulating and encouraging
- Divergent thinking and encouraging the other to be creative

- Problem solving
- Decision making
- Changing behaviour and developing skills
- Maintaining behaviour
- Knowledge of resources
- Evaluating

We would argue that all nurses need the skills facilitating exploration (Stage I), many nurses need the skills facilitating understanding (Stage II) and those nurses whose work brings them regularly into more formal counselling relationships need the skills facilitating action (Stage III). Many of the problems nurses have to help other people with are at the level of Stage I or II.

Consider, for example, the young woman who is confused about her reactions to her new baby. She may need some help in sorting out her conflicting feelings about her baby. This might be enough. Similarly, the middle-aged woman who is overweight and needs a hip replacement may need help in clarifying her feelings too, but may also need help in seeing what her refusal to diet is doing to herself and her family in terms of her increasing dependence on them to get about.

As understanding increases it can lead to decisions relating to how different strategies and lines of action might turn out. These can lead us to further explorations which in turn can lead to new insights and understanding and so on.

Consider, for example, the young man who has a spinal cord injury from a swimming accident. He can no longer walk or carry on any sporting activities. He cannot see how he will develop any interests or get to meet new people. He is convinced no one would want to be friends with him because he is wheelchair-bound. For this young man, exploration, understanding and alternative courses of action are all indicated, reflecting each stage of the counselling model.

We have seen, then, that nurses often have to use counselling skills in helping their patients, and those that are most frequently called for are those associated with Stages I and II of the counselling model. We will go on to consider these skills in some detail.

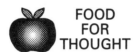

FOOD FOR THOUGHT

When is it enough to 'stop' at the exploration stage?

How do we know when understanding has been reached?

What factors inhibit nurses from encouraging patients and relatives to explore complex problems?

What is the role of colloquial expressions in communicating feelings?

How do children talk about different feelings?

How do we talk about our feelings to our parents or grandparents?

What geographical differences are there in ways of talking about feelings?

Skills facilitating exploration

These skills are the most basic and indispensable of the counselling skills and can be used to good effect in many different nursing contexts. Many have already been discussed as they overlap considerably with 'facilitation' skills. Effective use of questions is essential for helpful listening (Burnard, 1989). Listening, in counselling, is often an active process. It goes beyond attending to and receiving the message and extends to communicating to the speaker that the facts and feelings have been heard and that the person is understood. **Paraphrasing**, **reflecting** thoughts and feelings and **summarizing** are all ways in which nurses can indicate that they understand, accept and empathize (Dickson, 1986). Empathy is the ability to put ourselves in other people's shoes, to see a situation as if we were within their frame of reference. Non-verbal behaviour can indicate interest and attention, both necessary components of empathy. However, verbal skills are also required to convey our understanding to others.

We need a variety of words representing different feelings and strengths of feeling if we are to express our understanding accurately. Nurses meet people from different social groups and ethnic backgrounds, all of whom may have different colloquial expressions relating to bodily functions, medical procedures and emotional states. Paraphrasing and reflecting are two skills that help to communicate empathy. To paraphrase is to put what someone has said in different words without losing the essence of the original statement. Thus the use of synonyms and metaphors is required. It is useful to understand the colloquial forms of expression people from different generations and from different parts of the country use when describing their feelings and their illnesses. Reflection is a form of paraphrasing that is generally limited to feelings. The purpose is to take all that another person says and to draw out the feelings contained therein both to show understanding and acceptance and to clarify them for that person.

Consider, for example, the practice nurse talking with a woman who has received a report indicating that there is no more need for chemotherapy for a breast tumour.

Woman: When I got the results I felt on top of the world – no more tests and samples.
Practice nurse: I think you mean you were thrilled the results mean no more treatment. (*paraphrasing*)
Woman: Yes, I was.

Similarly:

Woman: When I got the results I felt on top of the world – no more tests and samples.
Practice nurse: It seems you were pleased. (*reflection*)
Woman: Yes.

In both these examples the patient confirms that the nurse has picked up her feelings correctly. Had she not done, the woman would have been able to correct her understanding or to elaborate.

> She might say at the end of one of the above exchanges, for example:
>
> **Woman**: Yes – but most importantly it means I can now go on holiday as planned. My husband was so looking forward to it.

Paraphrasing and reflecting are, then, skills that are essential for Stage I of the counselling model. These skills may seem strange at first, but with practice they will become more natural.

To help others explore their problems, active listening is vital. It is, however, sometimes not enough, and the skills of **focusing** and of **moving conversations on** have to be used, to encourage others to clarify their central concerns. Focusing may be used when people reveal complex concerns, with the different parts all mixed up, or when they make very general sweeping statements. Focusing helps them clarify and be more specific. The list below outlines some ways of moving conversations on by summarizing what has been said in different ways.

Some methods of summarizing to move conversations on (from Kagan, Evans and Kay, 1986)

At various stages during a helping interview with another person it may be necessary to try to move the interview on. Summarizing can help to do this. Summarizing can also help end a lengthy interview and create a 'set' or expectation about the issues to be considered on a subsequent occasion.

Summarizing using a contrast
The summary includes a paraphrase of the issues and a suggestion that the speaker considers some alternatives that might be available, e.g.,

> You must have had a very unhappy time in hospital. I wonder, though, if you could look ahead and think how you'd feel if you just walked out, now, in the middle of your treatment.

Summarizing using a choice point
The summary includes a paraphrase of the issues and a suggestion

that the speaker thinks about the various concerns and chooses one to work on, e.g.,

> You must have had a very unhappy time in hospital. There seem to be several things that are bothering you – not know- ing what's wrong with you, worrying about dying young as both your parents did and getting angry at the lack of con- sideration of the nursing staff. I guess we'll need to explore them all. Which do you think we should start on?

Summarizing using figure-ground, i.e., identifying the uppermost issue
The summary includes a paraphrase of the issues and a sugges- tion of which issue may be of the greatest concern, e.g.,

> You must have had a very unhappy time in hospital. There seem to be several things that are bothering you – not know- ing what's wrong with you, worrying about dying young as both your parents did and getting angry at the lack of con- sideration of the nursing staff. It feels as if your fear of dying is causing you most concern just now. I wonder if it would be useful to talk about that a bit more.

In this section we have briefly discussed some foundation counsel- ling skills that help others explore their problems in order to bring about greater clarity. We will now go on to consider some of the skills that are required for Stage II of the counselling model (Figure 9.1), namely those skills that facilitate understanding.

Skills facilitating understanding

The skills that facilitate understanding help people who have problems see things more objectively and form new perspectives, as well as helping them to increase their self-awareness and set themselves (appropriate) goals (see list above). We have considered some of these skills earlier (for example, self-disclosure, in Chapter 7), and all those discussed above are relevant too. In Stage II of the counselling model people with problems are challenged so that they develop greater understanding of their problems and of acceptable goals towards which to aim.

These techniques usually emerge in the course of a helping relation- ship and, as a rule, they should not be used in the exploratory stage, where non-directive skills are of more value. It is worth practising

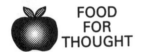

**FOOD
FOR
THOUGHT**

How easy is it to identify a) our own and b) other people's strengths?

How easy is to tell a) someone you do not know very well, b) your partner or close friend and c) a child what you think of as their strengths?

In what ways does nursing encourage you to identify and build on your strengths?

How does culture affect our willingness to discuss our strengths?

What difficulties arise when we try to set personal goals?

Are goals more easily set in some spheres of life than others?

some of these skills, as nurses frequently do develop helping relationships that extend over a period of time.

The overall aim of helping people understand their problem(s) is to enable them to set themselves realistic goals that they can go on to achieve. To be realistic, goals should be:

- concrete or specific rather than vague;
- clear and easy to recognize when they have been reached;
- within a person's scope and capabilities;
- within a person's values;
- attainable over a reasonable period of time.

It can be useful to think of goals in terms of the ways they form hierarchies. General goals lead to more specific goals and so on. Figure 9.2 illustrates a goal hierarchy.

There are two ways goal hierarchies (or goal trees) can be used to help people to greater understanding. The first is by **problem reduction**. This is the thinking through process illustrated in Figure 9.2. A general goal is identified and then questions are asked to encourage the person to 'unpack' the general goal into more specific, more concrete goals, ending up with specific actions that can be carried out.

The second technique is known as **laddering**. Laddering is the process of growing goal hierarchies, and is particularly useful when we

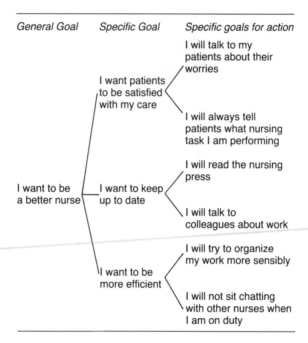

Figure 9.2 A goal hierarchy (from Kagan, Evans and Kay, 1986).

want to clarify why a particular goal is important. Once we have clarified this we may be able to come up with different alternatives for satisfying higher level goals.

Consider, for example, the colleague who wishes to introduce a new procedure in managing caseloads in the community. If we ask her why she wants to do this she may say it is because the change would encourage the team to discuss practice issues together. If we ask why she wants the team to work better and more supportively she may say it is to ensure the best patient care. If we ask why she wants the best patient care she might not have any further explanations other than 'because that is why we are in nursing'. We might have hit upon one of her highest level goals. The process is illustrated as follows:

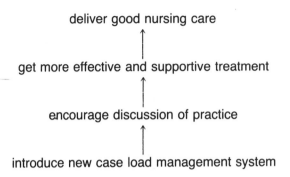

At this point it is possible to work back down the goal tree, asking in what ways the higher level goals might be satisfied. This process might produce more goals than the one that began the process, and goals that might be more suitable.

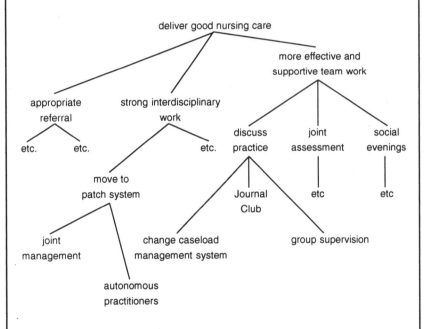

If nothing else, we may have clarified how the goal that has been set relates to other possible goals.

Having reached the stage of better understanding and the setting of goals, the issue remains of acting in such ways that goals can be met. This brings us to the helping skills that facilitate action.

Skills facilitating action

Nurses have, perhaps, less need of these skills than of those facilitating exploration and understanding. We have examined the social problem-solving process elsewhere (Chapter 5) but it is also relevant here. Some Stage III skills are too specialized to be included here (such as those of behaviour change and maintenance) and it is likely that few nurses other than those who work with people with either mental health problems or learning disabilities will have much call for them. However, we think that some of the techniques that encourage divergent thinking and that help reflect on barriers to change may be useful for nurses working in both hospital and community settings.

In thinking about different ways that a person may act for a change, it can often be helpful to 'brainstorm' ideas or possibilities. Brainstorming is a technique whereby one or more person(s) think(s) of as many associated ideas as they can, without rejecting any. Some of the ideas will be conventional, some unusual and some wildly impossible. Brainstorming is a means of thinking creatively about a problem and arriving at ideas for solutions that might be unusual, but possible. It is a way to help people think more broadly about possible courses of action at times when they would otherwise be stuck for alternatives.

When we help others consider and take various courses of action for themselves, it can help to examine with them some of the barriers that might impede their progress, so they can be realistic in their expectations of success or otherwise. Force-field analyses (see Stewart, 1983; Pfeiffer and Jones, 1974) are a tool to help us take an overall look at what helps or hinders progress towards a goal, and is illustrated in Figure 9.3.

In counselling, force-field analyses help people see how they could decrease hindering forces and increase and strengthen facilitating forces.

It is essential that progress and change is evaluated, and this can be described as the last skill of helping. Evaluation may indicate that further help or counselling is required or it may indicate that the problem is 'solved'. It is the person who originally sought help who must evaluate the outcome of that help in relation to her/his problem(s). It is the helper, though, who has the responsibility to summarize and check with the other person what has been achieved at various points throughout the counselling process.

So far in this chapter we have not considered the role of self-awareness. Perhaps more than in any other context, self-awareness is vital if nurses are to adopt counselling roles (Burnard, 1989; Macleod Clark, Hopper and Jesson, 1991; Tschudin, 1982). If we do not develop our own self-awareness, our own values and attitudes, fears and con-

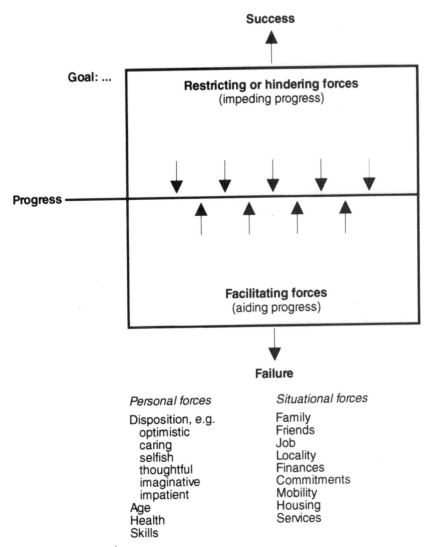

Figure 9.3 Force-field analysis (from Kagan, Evans and Kay, 1986).

cerns may well interfere with our ability to help others in ways that are as non-intrusive as possible. Thus the chapter on self-awareness (Chapter 2) is also of vital importance for the development of counselling skills.

We have not been able, in the space available, to explore counselling in any depth. Instead we have sought to select those skills that are of most relevance for nurses as helpers and sometimes as counsellors.

Consider, for example, the elderly woman with terminal cancer who has been living with her daughter but now wants to return to her own home 'to die'. There are many difficulties involved in this, and the district nurse has been helping her explore her concerns and arrive at a definite course of action. They have explored the issues and the elderly woman has decided her goal **is** to go home. What are the pressures or forces that might impede a successful return home? What are the forces that might help her successfully return home? We can set out the questions as follows:

Goal: to return home

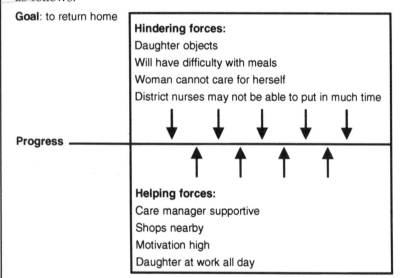

The task is to find things that will boost the helping forces and weaken the hindering or restraining forces. So, for example, a creative care package will strengthen the helping forces and assist in convincing the daughter that it is what her mother wants, and will weaken the hindering forces.

SUMMARY

This chapter has been concerned with some of the essential components of counselling skills. Specifically, the following points were raised.

- Counselling is a form of helping wherein one person enables another to engage in constructive resolution of personal problems.
- Counselling is a special form of helping and different in kind from persuasion, reassurance, advice, guidance and sympathy.
- Counselling enables other people to find solutions of their own after fully exploring their thoughts, feelings and behaviours.
- A person-centred approach to counselling seeks to create a trusting atmosphere in which others feel accepted, understood and valued.
- Counselling aims to help others reach a clearer understanding and to find their own strengths in order to make appropriate decisions.
- Counsellors support and encourage alternative ways to act and help others evaluate the consequences of their actions.
- Nurses are able to make use of counselling skills even if they rarely develop long-term counselling relationships.
- A warm and trusting atmosphere is a prerequisite of helping.
- An eclectic approach to the counselling process can be viewed in terms of three stages: exploration, understanding and action.
- Specific skills relate to different stages of the counselling process, although later stages incorporate skills of earlier ones.
- Many nurses can make good use of skills facilitating exploration and understanding and fewer can use those facilitating action.
- Skills relating to different stages of the counselling process may be used concurrently.
- Skills facilitating exploration help develop a warm relationship, communicate empathy and help the other person focus on specific issues.
- Verbal and non-verbal skills are essential if empathy is to be communicated.
- Skills facilitating understanding help people who have problems see things more objectively and from new perspectives as well as enabling them to set realistic goals for themselves.
- Reflection, paraphrasing and summarizing are all skills that can help people gain insight and communicate empathy.
- Active listening, focusing and the ability to move conversations on help people towards greater understanding.
- Goal setting is an important feature of personal understanding.
- It is useful to distinguish between general and specific goals.
- Problem reduction and laddering are two techniques that can increase people's understanding.
- Skills facilitating action help people plan and carry out courses of action in order to attain their goals.
- Force-field analysis is a problem solving method that examines the restraints on movement towards specified goals so that they can be decreased.

- Evaluation and checking are essential throughout the counselling process.
- Self-awareness in the counsellor is vital for effective helping.

SELF-DEVELOPMENT EXERCISES

1. Think of a time when someone else helped you with some personal difficulty you had. What was it about the way they acted or what they said that helped? Would the same things have helped in different circumstances? What kinds of helping do nurses most often engage in? Why is this?
2. With a friend, take it in turns to encourage each other to talk about an experience you have had (it does not have to be a traumatic experience – going for a walk in the country, for example, would be a suitable topic). Use active listening skills and questions to help each other discuss aspects of the experience you have not thought about, such as your feelings and sensations. Discuss the value of different kinds of question as an aid to exploration.
3. Collect a list of all the different expressions used to describe feelings that you come across in one week. Note which expressions are used by professionals, which by lay people and which you come across on television or radio. Think about the functions of colloquial expressions and how they might come about.
4. Paraphrase the following statements, taking care to identify the strength of feeling and the reasons for it.
    - I learned a lot in my last job and I now have a lot of experience behind me. Yes, I know my stuff with respect to surgical procedures and could face up to anything that happened there. The principles of medical nursing are the same, of course, although I am surprised at some of the practices here – standards don't seem to be the same. The staff are quite pleasant and most of them are interested in their work. Some have been here a long time. I'll be all right; I'll show them my ways.
    - (A middle-aged woman arrives at the ward to collect the belongings of her mother who died in the night:) Well, I'd like to say thank you for everything you've done – you've all been absolutely wonderful. We're both very grateful, my husband and myself. It was all very sudden; we didn't visit last night – Mother never seemed to want to talk – but then, of course, she wouldn't know if we'd been or not. We're both working such long hours, and I've been minding my grandchildren. I know we've no need to worry. You nurses are wonderful – she was a good patient, I know. She was in good hands.
    - I've not visited this patient before. Jim always describes her be-

haviour as unpredictable. Still, I've got lots of experience handling difficult people. I'm not sure what to do if she won't let me in. She'll have to have her injection – I can't get into the situation Barry found himself in when he was doing holiday cover. You know – couldn't get in, patient deteriorated and had to be admitted as an emergency. Trouble is, we build up such good relationships with our own patients, they don't trust anyone else.

5. Watch an audience participation programme on television concerned with current affairs (such as *Question Time*, *Kilroy*, *The Oprah Winfrey Show*, etc.). Imagine you are the presenter. Each time someone speaks, construct a reflection of what they have said. See if this tallies with the reflection offered by the presenter. As the programme goes on, try to summarize people's points in a way that would make them think of another perspective or issue. How easy is it to do this? Are some points that people make easier to summarize than other? What is the difference between those that are easy to summarize and those that are not? (You might find it helpful to video the programme before beginning this exercise, so you can pause the action while reflecting each speaker.)

6. Try summarizing the following scenarios and end directing the person in a particular direction for further thought and exploration.

   - You are a staff nurse in the community, talking with Anne Watson, who cares for her husband who is severely incapacitated by motor neurone disease. She has helped him now for 10 years with community staff help. She tells you that her two teenage daughters, who used to be so helpful, are now only concerned with going out and having a good time. They refuse to do their homework and will not bring friends home. Her husband is very weak and often will not get up. She is worried about his further deterioration. She begins to cry, saying she wants to run away and leave it all, and that her life is not worth living. She is still young and has lots to do in life.

   - You care for baby Angela on the neonatal intensive care unit. She was born at 26 weeks gestation and is surviving on major life support systems. Her parents have visited less in the last week. Next time her mother comes, she asks you why it is that Angela is put through so much suffering and says that if she does survive she won't live a normal life.

   - You work as a staff nurse in a private elderly persons' home. Amy Baxter (80 years old) has recently moved in. She is lively and interesting with a loving and attentive extended family. She goes visiting one or other of her family every weekend. Lately she has become quiet. You find out she regrets her decision to sell her beautiful home and come and be cared for. She does not want to burden her family, but feels her intellect will go if she spends much more time in the company of all these very old, apathetic people. She is despondent about the future and says she feels useless.

7. With a friend, discuss your future plans. Try to construct a goal hierarchy in relation to these plans. How easy is it to ladder up or down your hierarchy?

8. Identify, with a friend or colleague, a problem you face in relation to any aspect of your life. Identify the helping and hindering forces contributing to this problem. Talk through ways of strengthening or increasing the helping forces and weakening or reducing the hindering forces. Identify specific courses of action that you could take to try to resolve your particular difficulty. Discuss with your partner difficulties of carrying out a force-field analysis.

CHAPTER 10

Conflict, aggression and violence

Nurses have to deal with a range of interpersonal situations that contain conflict, verbal or physical aggression and sometimes violence. Their skills in these situations can be used in ways that lead to positive and constructive outcomes for all concerned. On the other hand, lack of skill can lead to the escalation of bad feeling or aggression.

HANDLING CONFLICT

Interpersonal conflict is usually thought of as destructive and damaging to good working relationships. Certainly poor communication, interpersonal disagreements and clashes can be harmful and demoralizing and lead to inefficiency at work. On the other hand, properly managed, conflict can be an energizing and vitalizing force. Schmidt (1974) identified both positive and negative outcomes of conflict from a survey of managers who spent about 20% of their time dealing with conflict situations. Table 10.1 outlines the positive and negative outcome of conflict.

Perhaps the best way to think about conflict is that it is never good or bad. It is, however an inevitable feature of life in complex organizations. Nurses, whether they are practice nurses in a small health centre, community psychiatric nurses working with people in a day centre, paediatric nurses working in a large hospital, or theatre nurses, all work in complex organizations within which conflicts, at personal, interpersonal, group or organisational levels will emerge.

Personal conflicts arise when people do not know what they want, are unable to make decisions or do not know how to achieve goals they have set themselves. Sometimes their personal goals may compete with each other, or a person may simultaneously want and not want to do something.

People experiencing internal conflict may need help to resolve the conflict from, for example a counsellor. Interpersonal group or organiz-

Table 10.1 Positive and negative outcomes of conflict

Positive outcomes	Negative outcomes
Long-standing problems revealed	Some people feel demeaned
Stimulation of interest and creativity	Distance between people is increased
Joint solutions found (if conflict is acknowledged)	Climate of mistrust and suspicion
Better and new ideas produced	Individuals and groups focus on own narrow interests
Clarification of individual views	Resistance encouraged
New understanding develops	Staff turnover
	Signs of stress

Consider, for example, the school nurse who is thinking of applying for a post as nurse for a large student hall of residence. She may both want to go and want to stay. She likes the children in the schools she works in but also likes the prospect of getting to know students. She is experiencing what is known as **approach–approach conflict**. However, the same nurse who gets offered the new job, but at a lower salary, may experience a different kind of conflict. Now she wants the job because of the new challenges it presents but she does not want the job because of the poor pay. She now experiences **approach–avoidance conflict**. To resolve either form of conflict she will have to make a decision, either by prioritizing some aspects of the old or new job; looking at the net costs or gains she would have in the new or old job, and so on.

ational conflicts arise when individuals (or groups) want different things and behave in incompatible ways.

If any of these conflicts are to lead to constructive outcomes they must be managed well by all concerned. Interpersonal and group conflicts cannot be managed solely by those in management positions, externally. Those involved in the conflict must take some part in its resolution.

Consider, for example, the mental health service of a community trust that is coterminous with a social services department. The community nurses may want to take direct and self-referrals and decide their own pattern of work and its priorities. The hospital consultants want the nurses to work to and for them, but they work primarily for the **hospital** trust, not the community trust. Nevertheless they continue to instruct the community nurses to attend particular ward rounds and nurse their patients. Some of the nurses would like to be 'attached' to consultant psychiatrists and others would not. GPs expect the nurses to be available as and when required. GP fundholders expect to be able to contract for new services with the nurses that have not hitherto been offered. Social service care managers, too, expect the nurses to deliver services that have not hitherto been offered.

We can see enormous potential for conflict here: between different groups of nurses; between nurses and psychiatrists; between different categories of GP; among purchasers from health, purchasers from social services and the nurses; and so on. Individual nurses would be confronted by colleagues who might or might not share the same aims and preferences. Sometimes the activities of some stakeholders might undermine those of others.

Styles of conflict resolution

People have different preferred styles of dealing with conflict. Some of these are more constructive than others and some are more likely to occur in some situations than others. Maddux (1988) suggests five common ways of resolving conflict, along with the justifications given for using them (Table 10.2).

The five ways of resolving conflict – avoidance, accommodation, win/lose, compromise and problem solving – differ in terms of assertiveness and co-operation. Each strategy can be mapped on to these dimensions, as shown in Figure 10.1.

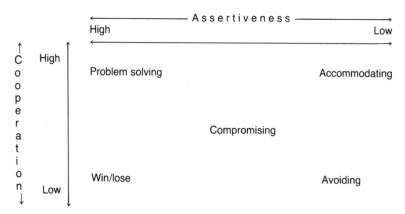

Figure 10.1 Methods of conflict resolution in terms of assertiveness and cooperation.

Some people may use strategies that are a mixture of styles and be located in an empty part of the grid shown in Figure 10.1. Our strategies may vary according to the situation and to the people with whom we are in conflict. Whatever the situation or role relationships between stakeholders, the most constructive strategies will be those

Table 10.2 Reasons for using different strategies for conflict resolution (adapted from Maddux, 1988)

What reason is given?	How is conflict resolved?	What is the style?
'Our differences are too minor or too great to resolve. Any attempt to do so may damage our relationship or create even greater problems'	Non-confrontational. Ignores or passes over issues. Denies issues are a problem	Avoiding
'It's not worth risking any damage to relationships or disharmony'	Agreeable, non-assertive. Cooperative with the sacrifice of personal goals or preferences	Accommodating
'The strongest person wins. I'm better and I'll prove it. I'm right and do what I'm expected to do as a nurse; others do not meet these standards'	Confrontational, assertive and aggressive. Must win at any cost	Win/lose
'We've all got faults. No-one's idea is perfect. There are different ways of doing things. We all have to give and take'	Endeavours to ensure everyone achieves their goals and maintain good relationships. Cooperative	Compromising
'When everyone will openly discuss things a mutually beneficial solution can be found to everyone's advantage'	Balances needs of all stakeholders. Respectful and supportive. Assertive and cooperative	Problem-solving

high in assertiveness and co-operation (that is, the problem-solving and compromise strategies).

If conflicts are poorly handled and not resolved they may escalate into aggression and even violence.

AGGRESSION AND VIOLENCE

There are many situations where nurses have to handle conflict, aggression and violence. They may experience conflict that merges into aggression with colleagues; conflicts that merge into verbal or physical aggression with relatives; and conflicts that merge with verbal or physical aggression and even violence with patients and some relatives. The ways nurses handle these incidents may exacerbate them and contribute to their escalation, or they may defuse them (Owens and Ashcroft, 1985; Maynard and Chitty, 1979).

Consider, for example, a staff nurse working in an accident and emergency department. A father brings his nine-year-old daughter in. She has received approximately 20 bee stings and is screaming. The department is very busy with six people from a serious road traffic accident being dealt with. Although there is a small notice explaining the triage system on the wall, the father knows nothing about it. He is agitated and requests his daughter be seen immediately by a doctor. The nurse begins to explain the priority system in terms of whether people are emergencies or not. She says it will be at least half an hour before a doctor will come. Soon after, another four people injured in a serious road traffic accident arrive. They are rushed into resuscitation cubicles. Eventually the nurse goes to the father and says it is now unlikely they will be seen for two hours. He gets very angry and shouts abuse about being a taxpayer and not getting what he's entitled to. The nurse tells him to quieten down as there are seriously ill people in the cubicles who have had to have emergency treatment. With this he pushes her against the wall and leaves, shouting that his daughter too is an emergency. As they pass, the daughter kicks the nurse screaming that she is an emergency.

This incident began with conflict, based on a mixture of emotional arousal and misunderstanding on the father's behalf, and a failure to explain procedures clearly on the nurse's behalf. Over time the father's and daughter's agitation increased. He perceived that his daughter was not getting the attention she needed and that others were jumping the queue. The nurse's explanation did not pacify him and eventually he became abusive and aggressive. So did his daughter.

The aggressive behaviour sequence

The example illustrates a number of important things about the nature of conflict, aggression and violence. Conflict, aggression and violence may all be part of a continuum, representing different intensities of the same thing. Goldstein and Keller (1986) describe the aggressive behaviour sequence. If strengths of feeling can be weakened at earlier stages in the continuum, later, more intense behaviour may be averted. Figure 10.2 illustrates the aggressive behaviour sequence.

This sequence is a useful one to understand in the context of people who may find it difficult to exert a great deal of self-control. The behaviour of some people with learning disabilities, for example, who are said to have 'challenging behaviour' (that is behaviour, sometimes of a physically demanding or violent nature, that challenges existing services) also follows this progressive sequence. If community nurses are able to defuse the intensity of expression at the weaker end of the continuum the more violent behaviour may lessen. Goldstein and Keller suggest that different intervention may be required in order to work with people who repeatedly reveal express behaviour at different points of the continuum.

The role of arousal

The case illustration also draws attention to another key issue in understanding aggression, namely the role played by physiological arousal. Berkowitz (1969, 1983) suggested that when people are thwarted they become frustrated. Of course, what people experience as frustration varies. Frustration leads to physiological arousal (increased adrenaline, heart rate, etc. – the flight–fight response). If the person labels this arousal as anger, and there is a suitable target in the environment, aggression may be expressed towards it. The process is illustrated in Figure 10.3.

However, the father in our example may also have considered that it was his turn to be allocated a scarce resource (the doctor). Ethological perspectives on aggression stress the importance of interpersonal competition for things that matter in understanding aggression (Lorenz, 1963).

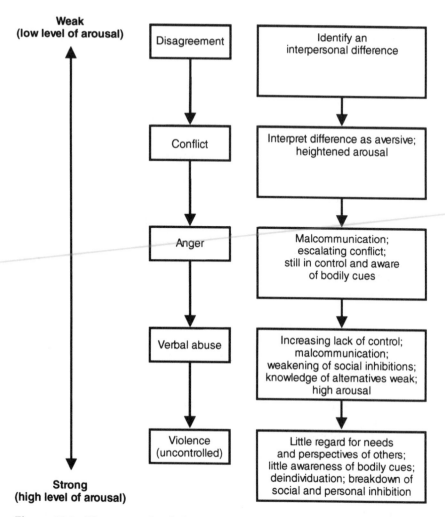

Figure 10.2 The aggressive behaviour sequence (after Goldstein and Keller, 1986).

Sometimes, the ways in which people have learnt to express their anger and aggression lead to particular ways of behaving. Social-learning theorists would suggest that this learning history is the key to understanding aggression (Bandura, 1977). From this perspective, it is essential to understand the antecedents (what went before), the aggressive behaviour and the consequences (what happened after). Indeed, this way of thinking mirrors the recommendations French (1983) makes for working with aggression. He argues that nurses should consider, and have strategies for dealing with, the prevention of an aggressive incident, the incident itself and aftercare. Thus picking

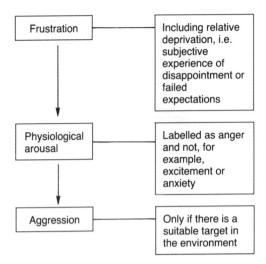

Figure 10.3 The frustration – aggression process in the context of individual interpretations.

up the signs of escalating aggression, handling the incident and support following an incident should all be part of nurses' interpersonal skill repertoires. Crossland (1992) goes further from this. In devising a training course for nurses in handling aggression (at any point in the aggressive-behaviour sequence) she highlighted the importance of nurses' self-awareness and competence in monitoring and using different ways of talking to people. In the course of having an aggressive incident, nurses reported feelings of arousal and anger themselves. By developing greater self awareness they were able to identify and manage their own escalating feelings and behaviours and thereby more effectively handle aggressive behaviours.

In a general discussion of aggression in different social situations, Kagan (1991) mentions a number of other things that are relevant to aggression in nursing situations. These include:

- the presence of other people at the scene of a potentially violent episode, which can lead to violence;
- the ways in which aggression may be used by some people in order to gain power or control over a situation;
- the ways in which the mass media either gives people ideas which they then copy in similar situations, or lowers the overall inhibition of aggression by making aggressive acts so commonplace;
- the different stressors in the environment (such as excessive heat, noise or crowds) which can catalyse aggression;
- The impact of de-individuation, whereby people's sense of self and individuality weaken, on the potential for people to be aggressive;

- the role of ritual and interpretation of events in aggression;
- the ways in which groups identify with their own members and have potential for conflict with other groups.

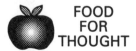

FOOD FOR THOUGHT

Are patients who are in their nightclothes during the day more irritable than those in their day clothes (the former are more de-individuated than the latter)?

Do strong and effective work teams cooperate well with other teams?

Are patients in the waiting room of a clinic more or less likely to express annoyance if there are other people in the waiting area?

Which perspective on aggression is able to explain why more men are violent than women?

How irritable are staff and patients when wards are very hot?

Why is aggression more likely when people are upset?

How might nurses help people reinterpret situations and thus reduce aggressive potential?

While the above discussion has focused mostly in ways to understand aggression, most nurses will meet many more instances of conflict and disagreement than they do of aggression and violence. Many of the verbal strategies used to handle conflict are those of assertion (Chapter 8).

SUMMARY

This chapter has been concerned with the skills of conflict, aggression and violence. Specifically, the following issues were raised.

- Conflict can be an energizing and vitalizing force if it is properly managed.
- Conflict can lead to both positive and negative outcomes.
- Conflict is an inevitable feature of life in complex organizations.
- Conflicts may occur at personal, interpersonal, group or organizational levels.
- Personal conflicts in decision making may be approach–approach conflicts or approach–avoidance conflicts.

- Interpersonal conflicts may be due to competing aspirations or incompatible behaviour.
- Those involved in conflict are in the best position to resolve it.
- People have different preferred styles of conflict resolution.
- Styles of conflict resolution, including avoidance, accommodation, win–lose, compromise and problem solving, vary in terms of assertiveness and cooperation.
- Effective styles of conflict resolution depend upon the situation.
- Conflict is closely linked to aggression.
- Aggression is usefully seen as a sequence of increasingly strong acts.
- The aggressive behaviour sequence includes disagreement, conflict, anger, verbal abuse and violence.
- Different interventions for diffusing and handling aggression are suitable for different stages of the aggressive behaviour sequence.
- Aggression is usually accompanied by physiological arousal.
- If arousal is labelled as anger, and there are trigger cues in the environment, aggressive behaviour may follow.
- Aggression is targeted.
- It is useful to understand both the antecedents and consequences of aggression if it is to be avoided in the future.
- Nurses should devise strategies for dealing with prevention of aggression, handling aggressive incidents and aftercare for those who have experienced aggression or violence.
- Self-awareness and self-monitoring are key features of the ability to handle aggressive incidents.
- The presence of other people may make aggression more or less likely.
- Aggression is a means whereby people can gain power over others.
- Environmental stressors and perceived lack of control can lead to aggression.
- People who experience de-individuation are more likely to be aggressive.
- Rules, rituals and group identity all play a part in people's willingness to be aggressive.

SELF-DEVELOPMENT EXERCISES

1. Think of situations at work in which you have experienced conflict with colleagues, patients or relatives. Identify the strategy (problem solving, accommodating, aggressive, win–lose, compromising, avoidance) you most often use with: a) colleagues who are senior to you; b) colleagues who are junior to you; c) colleagues who are equal in status to you; d) patients; e) relatives. Why do you employ different strategies with different people in different roles?

2. In groups of three or four people with whom you feel comfortable, talk through conflict situations you have all a) handled well and b) handled badly. Describe as fully as you can the context, background and development of the conflict. What was the source of the conflict (for example, approach–approach, approach–avoidance, personal standards or beliefs, etc.)? Was conflict expressed verbally, non-verbally or both? Where did the conflict take place? What was your relationship with the people involved? What feelings were aroused as the conflict developed? Did you have any fantasies about what you would have liked to have done or said during the conflict situation? How was it resolved in the end? How did you feel after the event and with whom did you discuss your actions and feelings? How would you handle the situation differently another time?

3. Think of a situation where you have had a disagreement with someone at work or at home. What did you want out of the situation? On what basis were you willing to compromise? Did you know what the other person or people involved wanted out of the situation? How easy was it to know the basis on which they might have been willing to compromise? Did you know what your own 'bottom line' was in terms of compromise? How easy is it to recognize this bottom line and stick to it?

4. Draw a picture of your work situation, identifying individuals you work closely with and groups of people who have a stake in your work (for example, other professional groups, patients, relatives, etc.). Draw lines linking people and groups together where there is a similarity of interests or goal. Draw a zigzag line linking people and groups who have some dissimilarity of interests or goals (there may be both zigzag and solid lines linking the same people). Can you see from your picture where alliances in any professional dispute might form? How might these alliances be used to help resolve conflict at work?

5. Observe a public situation (for example, in a post office, library, shop) or a television programme where an argument is going on. What signs were there that the argument would begin? What verbal and non-verbal signs are there that the argument is getting more heated? If the argument is escalating, what impact is there for those involved and any onlookers? How do people round about react to the argument? How do you feel observing all this?

6. Identify a nursing situation in which a patient gets frustrated (this could be with the delay in getting a bedpan, the slowness of post-operative recovery, the inability to reach something by the bed, receiving the wrong meal, and so on). How does her/his behaviour change? How might s/he deal her/himself with increasing frustration? How is her/his frustration expressed? Who receives the brunt of her/his annoyance? Are some people more prone to losing their

temper than others? What contribution does nursing practice play in increasing the frustrations of patients?

7. Discuss with a colleague who works in a different nursing setting from you the role of personal identity, disinhibition and autonomy in the tendency to become angry or aggressive. Do patients in their own homes get as irritable or angry as patients in hospital? Are patients who are upset more easily angered than those who are not? How might you use this knowledge to design a training module for student nurses beginning to work with people with severe learning disabilities and aggressive behaviour in the community?

8. How would you deal with the following situations.

   • You are a primary nurse on a surgical ward. A young man aged 20 has been admitted for neurological observations via the accident and emergency department following an assault outside a pub. It has not been possible to contact his next of kin. Two young men arrive, saying they are his friends. They demand to see him and from the moment they arrive they shout abuse at staff at the entrance to the ward. They smell of alcohol. They start to move towards the ward and push you sideways as you try to talk to them.

   • You are working in the community and are visiting a young male patient who has mental health problems. His mother lets you in but does not allow you to talk to her son, taking you through to the kitchen instead. There she berates you and the rest of the community staff for your lack of understanding of her son, lack of skill and poor quality of care. Her son comes in during this tirade and becomes visibly agitated, asking his mother to stop.

   • You are a research nurse reporting back to a group of hospital- and community-based mental health workers the results of an evaluation study of a reorganized part of the service. One of the consultants starts to get angry. He stands up and shouts that he and his colleagues know how the service should be run and that they do not need a so-called researcher to tell them what to do. He shows no signs of stopping and everyone else begins to look very uncomfortable.

   • You are alone on a ward at night-time. A middle-aged female patient calls you over and suddenly gets out of bed, pulling out her intravenous lines as she does so. She sweeps the equipment off her locker and pushes you aside. She shouts that she is going home and that you are keeping her against her will. She storms out of the ward, knocking you into a table as she does so, clad only in her nightclothes.

CHAPTER 11

Social problem solving (2)

Nurses are increasingly having to deal with complex situations involving sensitive face-to-face interpersonal skills at times of distress and complex interpersonal skills with a range of different people in the context of organizational change. These two types of situation represent the ends of a continuum of interpersonal skills in which the social problem-solving process can be useful. The continuum is one of social complexity. Relatively simple social situations are those in which few people are involved and their reasons for being involved are quite clear. Complex situations are those in which very many people are involved and the nature of their involvement varies and may or may not be clear. The complexity of the situation is not defined in terms of the complexity of the issue under consideration. As we shall see, simple situations can involve highly complicated issues.

In this chapter we will take examples from the two types of situation and consider the place that social problem solving has in the interpersonal skills involved in working within each. The first section is concerned with breaking bad news. This is an example of a relatively simple situation. Generally there will not be very many people involved and their reasons for being involved are clear. There are those who are in a position to give bad news because of their role or expert knowledge and those who will receive the news because of their relationship and involvement in the medical or nursing issue at stake. The second section is concerned with some of the interpersonal skills involved in managing organizational change. This is an example of a complex situation as there are many different stakeholders, not all of whom will have much contact with nurses but whose interests need to be taken into account.

BREAKING BAD NEWS

Situations that entail the breaking of bad news occur frequently in nursing and will vary in the degree of trauma and upset that is involved. At one extreme nurses may be in the position of informing a patient about the negative outcome of a test, particular procedure or even a diagnosis. At the other extreme nurses may be in the position to tell colleagues about their unsuccessful job interview. In between these two examples may be many different situations where nurses are in the position of breaking bad news to patients, relatives or professional colleagues.

Whatever the situation, breaking bad news should be seen as part of a process that begins with exploration and preparation, identifies some outcomes and strategies by which they may be achieved and includes follow-up support or guidance. Different people may be involved at different stages and the ways in which the stages are handled may vary with the situation. The process of breaking bad news resembles the problem-solving process as shown in Table 11.1.

People's reactions to bad news vary and it is not always easy to predict how any particular person will react. However, the way people are prepared for bad news, the way it is actually broken and the quality of any follow-up support will all influence its impact.

In most circumstances affecting patients, nurses will either be present when distressing information is given by doctors, have a role in preparing patients to receive bad news at a later date or, perhaps most frequently, be the ones to provide support and further information after the news has been broken. There is a certain amount of evidence that in the absence of good postdiagnosis counselling and support, people can become anxious and depressed and in need of psychiatric support (Tait, 1985).

If nurses are unaware of their feelings about debilitating illness, disability, death and dying or failure of different sorts they are likely to use their interpersonal skills to block open communication or divert attention away from the issue. This in turn can give out strong messages that the issues should not be discussed.

Similarly, though, nurses in these situations need support themselves if they are to be able to carry on working in emotionally laden contexts (Yasko, 1983; Vachon and Lyall, 1976).

It can be useful to understand some of the reactions that some

Table 11.1 Breaking bad news as problem solving

Breaking bad news	Problem solving
Exploration and preparation	Perception
	Definition
Identification of outcome	Identification of goals
Strategy formulation	Generalization of alternatives
	Choice of solution
Course of action	Action
Reviews and follow-up	Evaluation

people have to loss – whether this is in the context of bereavement, health or achievement and loss. The loss may be current or it may be anticipated for some time in the future and thus the reaction may come during preparatory, breaking-the-news or follow-up periods. Not everyone will react to bad news in this way; indeed it is very difficult to predict in advance what is and is not bad news. It has been suggested (Parkes, 1972; Kubler-Ross, 1970, 1986; Lendrum and Symes, 1992) that people go through a number of stages in reacting to loss. Some people may need help in moving from one stage to another and this is the role of the bereavement counsellor. Having moved from one stage, people can return to an earlier one; the process of adjustment is not always linear. The stages suggested are shown in Table 11.2.

Nurses too have to adjust to loss and anticipated loss. If they are not prepared for this and have inadequate support systems, they may use a range of unhelpful interpersonal strategies. These include the following:

- denial of seriousness of person's condition;
- abrupt change of conversation;
- behaving as though person has not spoken (prevalent in relatives when patient is trying to express fears);
- intense concentration on legitimate task (e.g., writing prescription, engaging in nursing task/household duty, etc.);
- introducing a joking atmosphere;
- leaving the stressful situation;

Table 11.2 Stages of adjustment to significant loss (significant loss will vary from one person to another)

Stage	Feelings of
1. Numbness	Shock
	Disbelief
2. Yearning	Reminiscence
	Searching
	Hallucinating
	Anger
	Guilt
3. Disorganization and despair	Anxiety
	Loneliness
	Ambivalence
	Fear
	Helplessness
	Hopelessness
4. Reorganization	Acceptance
	Relief

- pursuing the least threatening aspect of the conversation;
- introducing a formal/professional manner (prevalent amongst medical personnel).

Part of the problem solving around breaking the news is personal problem solving, that is, identifying and finding solutions for personal difficulties arising from emotionally demanding nursing practice.

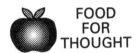

FOOD FOR THOUGHT

What news is bad news?

What assumptions do you make in thinking of these things as inherently bad?

What is the role of 'self' in thinking about whether a particular piece of medical news is good or bad?

Are some things easier to discuss with men or women?

Are some things more difficult to discuss with people of different ages or cultures? Why is this?

How does your personal experience influence the way you give different kinds of news?

What would it take to devise a policy within your work team relating to breaking the news?

Hacking (1981) suggests that nurses will often be asked those practical questions about death and dying (and indeed about the course of different medical conditions) that patients and their relatives are reluctant to raise with doctors. Often these discussions reveal deep-seated fears and anxieties. Hacking suggests a number of features of good practice applicable to different situations: attention and interest; time; a quiet place; relaxed and positive facial expression; comforting touch; when words are superfluous, appropriate silence; confidence and honesty.

The ways in which relatives are told of serious illness or disability can influence their relationships with each other. The potential damage that is possible can be illustrated by examples where problems at birth are dealt with clumsily and insensitively.

Dale *et al.* (1991) outline the main points to consider in breaking the news to parents that their child has a disability. (This will not necessarily be at birth, but may be when the child is considerably older.) They recommend:

Consider, for example, the situation of a newborn baby. The obstetrician present at the birth rushes the baby straight off to a special care baby unit. Twelve hours later the mother is permitted to see her. Meanwhile, as she puts it, 'the staff avoided me'. The baby has tubes up her nose and is blue. The doctor tells the mother she 'isn't feeding' and then asks 'Have you ever heard of Down's syndrome?' The mother just screams. She is told the baby has a heart defect and needs special care. Her husband comes to see her with a big bunch of flowers – he knows nothing about it. She is left on her own to tell him. Later on the paediatrician explains to the mother what the problem and the diagnosis is. The mother is so upset she doesn't hear. During her stay in hospital she is put in a side ward and feels isolated. She has no contact with nurses, who avoid her. It isn't until she gets home and is visited by a special care midwife that anyone sits down with her, listens to what she had to say and helps her see that she will be able to cope. Eventually she meets other parents who are able to give her support, both in caring for her daughter and in helping repair her damaged relationship with her husband. This baby remains part of the family – many do not.

- Tell the truth.
- Break the news gently and sensitively.
- Take it at the pace of the parent(s).
- Avoid degrading descriptions.
- Transmit hope.
- Write down the relevant information.
- Ask the parent(s) to draw up a list of questions.
- Offer to break the news to other relatives.
- Follow up with subsequent visits.
- Avoid 'We don't have the time' excuses.
- Give information on local resources.
- Keep parent(s) informed of all developments as soon as possible.
- Parent(s) may not resolve many conflicts while in hospital – it usually takes years.
- The degree of sensitivity, concern and respect for parents you manifest in this situation will greatly influence the productiveness of future working relationships between professionals and parents.

Good communication among members of the care team will ensure that patients, relatives and colleagues are given a consistent message by everyone involved in a particular instance and this can be vital, particularly if care is intended to be delivered in what Glaser and Strauss (1965) call an 'open awareness' context (see Field, 1984; Knight and Field, 1981).

MANAGING CHANGE

Change at a personal level has been discussed in Chapter 9. However, many nurses are increasingly required to manage interpersonal change. New roles have been created in recent years for, for example, clinical assistants (Caine, 1993; Bottom, 1987) and there have been massive organizational changes throughout the health service that have affected staff, patients and their relatives. Some of these changes have disrupted existing working relationships and others have created new ones. All the changes present interpersonal challenges to nurses that can be conceptualized as specific kinds of social problem and are, therefore, subject to the social problem-solving process.

Plant (1987) identifies six key activities for the successful implementation of change, as illustrated below.

Key activities for successful implementation of change

1. *Help individuals or groups face up to change*
- reward and encourage risk taking
- support and reinforce those who are positive
- keep everyone fully informed of progress

2. *Communicate like you have never communicated before*
- reduce uncertainty, secrecy and complacency
- feed information up and down the organization
- ensure information flow between work units
- use informal and formal channels

3. *Gain energetic commitment to the change*
- focus sharply on the importance of the change to the success of the unit or organization
- encourage a common vision about what could be (and what the alternatives might be without the change)
- frame explanations positively

4. *Ensure early involvement*
- involve all stakeholders
- give information
- encourage a sense of ownership

5. *Perceive change as opportunity*
- Encourage the perception of change as natural, continuing, and opportunity
- focus on the benefits that will come from change

6. *Avoid over-organizing*
- adopt flexible strategies
- be open to suggestion and information from all parties

These activities all depend for their success on the skills and acts of those trying to implement the changes. Most importantly those people who manage change effectively are acutely aware of themselves and others and can identify sources of resistance within and between people.

Consider, for example, the community nurse manager in a well integrated, multidisciplinary primary health care team. The area has a number of GP fundholders and an NHS community trust. Whereas in the past district nurses carried out assessments and planned care, they are now part of a provider unit. They must change their working relationships with (new) health and social services purchasers, as well as with their erstwhile social worker colleagues (most of whom are now care managers). The nurse manager has a major task in implementing the changes that have resulted from legislation. She may meet considerable resistance from nurses who do not like the new arrangements, are skilled in assessment, do not understand community care legislation, and so on. How is she to implement change in a constructive and beneficial way?

Much of the handling of the interpersonal aspects of change involves motivating and encouraging others to be involved and to view the change positively. Lack of motivation can be either a symptom or a cause of 'burnout' (see Chapter 14).

Some sources of motivation lie in the way nurses' jobs are structured. However, recognizing the contribution people make to their work and the wellbeing of their patients contributes to raised morale. On the other hand, failing to recognize these things can lead to low morale. Scott and Rochester (1984) identify a number of features of considerate interpersonal behaviour that are aspects of good leadership. While they might appear self-evident, nurses from a variety of settings will be able to attest to the fact that they are not always employed. They have wide relevance to all working relationships. The elements of considerate interpersonal behaviour are summarized below.

Considerate and constructive interpersonal behaviour

Communicate
Talk to each other often; share positive attitudes to the job; get to know each other; listen when others talk to you

Be courteous
Treat each other with respect and good manners

Be tactful
Do nothing hurtful or spiteful, let others save face; admit mistakes and accept blame as appropriate

Be tolerant
Suffer mistakes in others; accept people for what they are

Keep your temper
Recognize that losing temper is hurtful and will jeopardize good relationships

Praise and criticism
Express approval and appreciation and thanks when they are deserved; give praise when due but avoid flattery; be constructive in criticism; criticize the idea or the behaviour, not the person

Be sincere
Mean what you say; keep promises;

Be loyal
Do not criticize people behind their backs; defend people when necessary

Resistance to change

Whenever change is on the horizon or actually being implemented, some people will resist it. The reasons people might resist change vary, although Plant (1987) suggests that resistance is either systemic or behavioural. **Systemic resistance** arises from inappropriate knowledge, information, skills and management. **Behavioural resistance** derives from the reactions, perceptions and assumption of individuals and groups in the organization. Whilst systemic resistance can be dealt with by good management practice, consultation and information flows, behavioural resistance includes emotional reactions such as lack of trust and is therefore more difficult to deal with. It requires high levels of individual skills to be overcome.

One of the things that sometimes happens when nurses find themselves caught up in changes they do not fully understand (or may even think are wrong) is that they begin to feel unable to control events. As a result they may display **reactance** as a means of trying to regain control again (Wortman and Brehm, 1975). This process was illustrated in Figure 2.1. Reactance can appear as uncooperative, stubborn behaviour, often leading to the undermining or sabotage of change. Resistance to change is a natural phenomenon, but it is likely to be greater if levels of involvement and information are low. Table 11.3 outlines major sources of resistance to change and strategies used to overcome them.

Exactly the same case can be made in respect to patients. Illness and its treatment is a change process. If patients feel out of control they may well develop reactance as a means of regaining control. This can damage their recovery prospects and much has been said about the importance of information and participation as key components of good recovery (see, for example, Davis, 1985 and Robinson, 1989 for discussion of these two issues).

Many of the skills of working with others in the context of change overlap with those considered in the discussions of assertiveness (Chapter 8) and counselling (Chapter 9) and are also employed in the skills of supervision and appraisal (Chapter 13) and conflict management (Chapter 10)

SUMMARY

This chapter has been concerned with social problem solving in two different types of situation, breaking bad news and the management of change. Specifically, the following issues were raised.

- Breaking bad news is involved in many different types of nursing situation.

Table 11.3 Sources of resistance to change and strategies for overcoming them (see Mullins, 1989 for full discussion)

Sources of resistance		Strategies to overcome resistance
Individual resistance	*Organizational resistance*	
Selective perception	Preference to maintain stability	Early involvement and participation in key decisions
Habit	Investment in current resources	Information
Inconvenience or loss of freedom	Past contracts or agreements	Environment of trust and shared commitment
Economic implications	Threats to power or influence	Cooperative spirit among work teams
Past security	Past performance	Changes to work systems recognize people's skills and
Fear of the unknown	Misinterpretation	preferences
Reluctance to take risks		Development of cohesive work groups
Threat to skills and confidence		
Threat to status		
Strong peer group norms		

✗ ● Breaking bad news involves exploration, preparation, particular strategies, evaluation and follow-up.
● The process of breaking bad news parallels that of problem solving.
● People's reaction to bad news depends in large part on their preparedness to receive it.
● Nurses may not be responsible for giving the news itself but will have important parts to play in preparing and supporting people who receive it.
● Self-awareness is crucial to nurses' ability to be open and honest in giving bad news to others or supporting those who receive it.
● Some people may react to bad news in a similar way as to loss.
● Nurses need to find personal solutions to personal difficulties relating to emotional aspects of nursing.
● If bad news is given clumsily or in a misleading manner, patients' relationships and their ability to cope may be severely hampered.
● Nursing and medical teams should have established procedures and back-up for staff who may be involved in giving bad news.
● Successful implementation of change depends on the skills and acts of those in a position to implement change.
● Self-awareness is central to the ability to manage one's own and others' resistance to change.
● Skills of motivating and encouraging others are essential for successful management of change.
● The nature of nurses' work itself, during change, may affect motivation.
● Resistance to change may arise in the system or in individual people.
● Good management practice, consultation and information can reduce systemic resistance.
● Emotional support and understanding can help reduce individual resistance.
● Participation in the change process helps reduce individual resistance.
● Feelings of personal control are essential for constructive involvement in processes of change.

SELF-DEVELOPMENT EXERCISES

1. Think of the context in which you work. What is the policy about giving bad news, of whatever sort, to patients? Who gives the news? What back-up is there for staff working with the patient? Is the context an open or closed awareness context? What tensions does this context create for you?

2. How would you go about giving the following types of news:
   - as a ward manager, telling a new patient admitted for gynaecological surgery, who has travelled a long way and waited five hours for a bed, that none will be available today;
   - as a night nurse of a medical ward, going over the information a 32-year-old mother of four has been given about the poor prognosis of her leukaemia;
   - as a community nurse who visits the parents of an autistic young man (they will not talk to any other support staff, as they do not think the care their son receives is adequate) with the police in order to inform them that their son has been missing from his city centre home for eight hours;
   - as the staff nurse in an antenatal clinic who is present when a 42-year-old primigravida is told that the results of her amniocentesis test reveal that her unborn baby has Down's syndrome;
   - as the primary nurse who is asked to tell a confused 84-year-old patient, in hospital because of severe vitamin deficiencies, that her husband has died at home.
3. With a friend, talk about your reaction to the first death of a patient with whom you had a good relationship in your nursing career. What was your reaction? Can you identify different stages of coming to terms with her/his death? Were there any features of work or support from friends that helped you come to terms with it?
4. Imagine you are an internal consultant to your own place of work. Your brief is to design the best system for delivering bad news to patients and relatives. What would you include in this system and why?
5. Outline the changes that have taken place in your work. Include aspects of change in the following domains: personal, interpersonal, group, organizational and cultural. What do you think the primary change issue has been?
6. With a colleague, discuss a recent change that has been introduced at work. Identify the different stakeholders in the change and try to identify the interests of the different stakeholders in the outcome of the change. Did resistance to change take place? Identify resistance within the system and resistance offered by individual people. What impact did resistance have on the successful implementation of the change, and on your experiences of change? Discuss the possible reasons why you and your partner differ in your views of any part of the discussion.
7. Watch and listen to colleagues talking to each other during one week. Can you identify any constructive and considerate ways in which they treat each other? Why is this (do they understand each other, like each other, rely on each other, think in the same way as each other, and so on)?

8. Imagine you are an internal consultant to your place of work. Take any particular change project that is currently under way. How would you advise managers and staff on the best way of implementing the changes? What is it you are taking into account in offering this advice?

CHAPTER 12

Working with groups

Nearly all nurses work in and with groups at some point. Common nursing situations demanding group understanding and skill include:

- ward reports and ward rounds;
- ward management meetings;
- communal meal times for patients;
- some out-patient waiting rooms;
- team briefings and meetings, case conferences;
- joint supervision sessions, meetings with patients and relatives, visits to a family.

THE NATURE OF GROUPS

Whenever three or more people exert mutual influence on each other (either through face-to-face contact or from a distance) they are said to be a group.

The influence factor is important because not all collections of three or more people sharing time and space constitute a group. They may just be three or more people who are in the same place at the same time, not necessarily even for the same reason.

Consider, for example, 15 people waiting in out-patients for a clinic. They are there for the same reason so they share a common purpose. However, they are not interacting in any way. A nurse comes in and tells them there will be a further delay of almost one and a half hours as the doctor has been called away. Suddenly, there is a hubbub as people begin talking to each other and discussing their common plight. It could be said that they are now a group as they not only have a common purpose but also exert influence on each other (by talking). One young man is not joining in the discussions. He is thinking what his father, mother and grandmother would say if he talked to people he did not know. His mother and his father and his grandmother are what is known as a **referent group**. They are not present, but they still exert an influence on his behaviour.

However, it could be said that unless the people shared a common understanding of their group, i.e., they felt some group identity, they could not be considered a group just because they interacted or influenced each other's behaviour.

We can see from the above example that groups do not in fact exist. The term 'group' is an abstraction used to define particular forms of interpersonal behaviour and experience.

Behaviour and experience within groups fluctuates and group processes are known as **group dynamics** (Forsyth, 1983; Shaw, 1981).

It can be useful to distinguish between group structures and processes (Brown, 1988; Whittaker, 1985). We will consider here the group processes and structures of communication, roles, leadership, power, participation and empowerment, team development and multidisciplinary team work. Like most conceptual distinctions, structures and processes do not separate easily and there will be some overlapping.

COMMUNICATION IN AND BETWEEN GROUPS

Group performance and experience is influenced by the interactions between members of the group. This is in turn influenced by channels of communication. In face-to-face groups six different patterns of communication have been identified (Leavitt, 1951): these are the wheel, circle, 'Y', all-channel and two chains. Figure 12.1 illustrates these patterns.

The **wheel** is a centralized network with a key link-person through which communications are channelled. The **circle** is decentralized but not fully participatory, as is the **all-channel network**. **'Y'** and **chain networks** involve little interaction and may be indicative of poor group relationships or of simple group tasks.

These communication processes are partly dependent upon structure. Interaction is difficult if group members sit in a line or if some people cannot see or be seen. Similarly the types of chair people sit on and their relative heights if standing can influence ease of communication.

The amount people speak and the nature of their contributions affects the working of the group and the experiences of the members. In mixed sex groups, men (and boys) generally talk more than women (and girls). As a result they may begin to dominate the group and others may get bored or uninterested. In many groups both task-related and supportive (or socio-emotional) functions emerge in order to keep

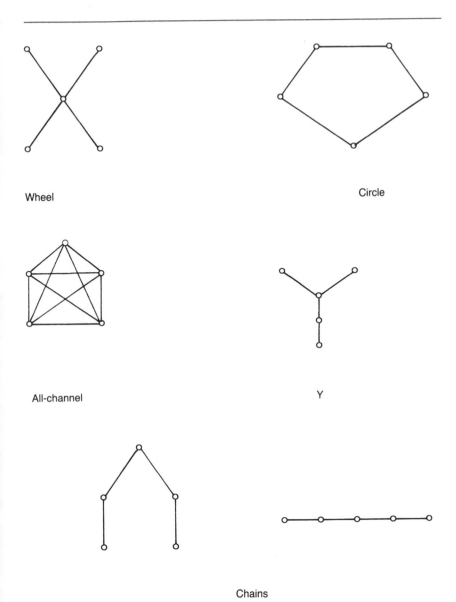

Wheel

Circle

All-channel

Y

Chains

Figure 12.1 Patterns of communication in five-member groups.

the group going to fulfil its purpose and satisfy its members. These two functions are often revealed through the content of what is said and how. Bales (1950) categorized every act in group discussion under 12 headings, differentiating between task and socio-emotional acts. The categories and acts are outlined as follows.

Interaction process analysis: observation Categories (after Bales, 1950)

Supportive: socio-emotional (positive)
- **Shows solidarity**: supports, rewards, enhances others' status, gives help
- **Shows tension release**: laughs, jokes, expresses satisfaction, distracts
- **Shows agreement**: passively accepts, understands, concerns, complies

Task: problem solving
- **Gives suggestion**: directs, sustains autonomy of others
- **Gives opinion**: evaluates, analyses, expresses feelings
- **Gives orientation**: informs, repeats, clarifies, confirms

Task: questioning
- **Asks for orientation**: informs, repeats, confirms
- **Asks for opinion**: evaluates, analyses, expresses feelings
- **Asks for suggestion**: directs, requests possible ways of acting

Unsupportive: Socio-emotional (negative)
- **Shows disagreement**: passively rejects, formal, withholds help
- **Shows tension**: asks for help, withdraws
- **Shows antagonism**: deflates others, defends or asserts self

These interaction categories have formed the basis of a system for analysing interaction process within groups, although it should be noted that some of the richness of quality of interaction is lost when it is reduced to 12 categories. Alternative approaches to group interaction are becoming more popular (Parker and Burman, 1993). Nevertheless, it is thought that task or problem solving aspects of group behaviour and maintenance behaviours – concerned with the feeling of group members – are useful ways to think about groups at work.

As group members meet and interact they adopt particular roles. Some of these may have been allocated in advance (such as chair, minute-taker); others will emerge as time goes on.

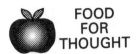

**FOOD
FOR
THOUGHT**

When carrying out a visit to a patient's home, how easy would it be to communicate if you were standing and the family were sitting?

When interviewing a new colleague, how would communication be affected if the four-member interview panel were all sitting on hard, high chairs and the interviewee was in a low, soft chair?

What difference does forming a circle make to communication in groups?

What is the optimum communication network for a case conference in which a key member speaks with the aid of a translator?

How do channels of communication change if a member of the group is visually impaired?

ROLES

It could be said that people who fulfil either task or socio-emotive functions also fulfil task or socio-emotive roles. However, most groups contain many more roles than these two. There are different roles associated with the tasks the group may have and the way it satisfies its members. There are also roles linked to individual people and the ways they interact with specific others. Common roles emerging in many work groups are shown below.

Common roles played by members of work groups (adapted from Benne and Sheats, 1948)

Individual roles	*Maintenance roles*	*Task roles*
The aggressor	(linked to the way the	The initiator
The blocker	group satisfies)	The opinion-giver
The critic	The encourager	The information-
The approval-seeker	The harmonizer	seeker
The help-seeker	The compromiser	The energizer

The know-it-all	The gate-keeper	The information-
The clown	The standard-setter	giver
The distracter	The observer/	The recorder
The belittler	commentator	The agenda/time-
The role-follower	The joker	keeper
	The positive thinker	

Any of these roles may be occupied by a formal or informal group leader. The important thing about exploring group dynamics in terms of role is that people behave, in part, according to other people's expectations. Thus, once someone plays the role of 'clown' in a group it may be difficult for her/him to be taken seriously and step out of this role. Similarly, once a role is occupied, other people may be reluctant to play it. Thus once a person occupies the role of compromiser, for example, other people may find it difficult to play this role on the occasion s/he is absent. By understanding the roles that are being played within a group we may also be able to understand the effectiveness of a group and the nature of communications. We will see later that a combination of different roles leads to effective work teams.

LEADERSHIP

A leader is a specific role that is played in groups. Leaders only exist alongside those that are led. Hersey and Blanchard (1988) argue that, while a great deal of research has been conducted into effectiveness of different leadership styles, it may well be the behaviour of the rest of the group that determines leader behaviour and thereby group effectiveness. Furthermore, the situations will change over time (Nicholls, 1985). Certainly, Fiedler (for example, 1976) proposed that effectiveness

Table 12.1 Leadership style and aspects of the situation (adapted from Fiedler, 1950)

Group atmosphere (inter-member relationships)	Task structure (clarity of purpose)	Position power (legitimation of leader)	Most effective leadership style
Good	High	Strong	Task-Oriented
Good	High	Weak	Task-Oriented
Good	Low	Strong	Task-Oriented
Good	Low	Weak	People-Oriented
Poor	High	Strong	People-Oriented
Poor	Low	Strong	People-Oriented
Poor	Low	Weak	Task-Oriented

of person-oriented or task-oriented leadership depended on the clarity and favourableness of the situation, the atmosphere between group members and the extent of legitimate power a leader has. Table 12.1 summarizes the link between leadership styles and other aspects of the situation.

Consider, for example, a primary health care team reorganized on a patch basis. The manager is a district nurse. The team is made up of several different nursing specialisms and professions, including health visitors, community mental handicap nurses, speech therapists (part-time), occupational therapists (part-time), orthoptists and chiropodists. The manager has high 'position power' – she has power by virtue of her position. However, she is new to the post and other team members do not consider her qualified to organize the team. This will weaken her position power. Most team members are unclear as to how the patch system is meant to work in the context of purchaser/provider arrangements although they are, in the main, a provider unit. They see little advantage in working as a team, as opposed to as specialist groups. The task structure is therefore weak. Furthermore, people have been redeployed into this patch team as a result of the reorganization and do not want to be there. Group atmosphere is not good.

All these circumstances will have to be taken into account when the team manager thinks about which style to adopt. A different set of circumstances might invite a different leadership style.

Adair (1983, 1984a,b) argues that in any work group the most effective leader is the person who sees that all the task needs, the needs of the group and those of individual members are met.

POWER

Leadership represents one type of power. Clearly other kinds of power accompany other roles and the balance of power can influence what goes on in the group. A well known way of looking at social power was offered by French and Raven (1959; French, 1964). They suggested that five main sources of social power could be identified. They all depend on the perceptions held by other people, and are all inter-related. Any one person may exercise different kinds of power in particular circumstances. The sources of social power are outlined below.

Sources of social power (after French and Raven, 1959)

Reward power
The perception that a person has the ability and resources to obtain rewards (such as pay, promotion, praise, recognition, allocation of duties, etc.)

Coercive power
Based on fear, the perception that a person has ability to punish (such as withholding performance related pay, prevention; formal reprimand; dismissal; allocation of undesirable duties; withdrawal of support, etc.)

Legitimate power
The perception that a person has a right to exercise influence by virtue of her or his position (such as manager, supervisor, employer, senior, anyone in authority, etc.)

Referent power
Identification as a result of perceived commonality (such as attractiveness, reputation, charisma, personal characteristics)

Expert power
The perception of a person as competent with specialist knowledge (e.g., in terms of nursing techniques, education and training, seniority, etc.)

Taylor (1989) reminds us that social power also comes from people's position in society. Power differentials exist along divisions in society such as race, sex, age, differential ability, and so on. When we consult with health service users or potential users we will often be inviting the least powerful citizens to meet on equal terms with some of the most powerful (that is, professionals).

Participation and empowerment

In some work groups power has been seen to be used destructively and to oppress those with least power from the start (Lukes, 1974). Indeed, when we think of how to encourage ordinary people to participate in care plans, case conferences, individual care reviews, we are faced with the problem of how to empower them to be equal participants along with professionals, but also, in the group meetings themselves, of how to ensure that they are given a powerful voice (Croft and Beresford, 1990; Thompson, 1991; White, 1988). This challenge is highlighted when we consider ways of enabling people who cannot speak for themselves (such as CVA survivors; non-English-speakers and people with learning disabilities) to participate in discussions and decisions about their health.

Some attempts to enable people to participate equally in groups have advocated removing existing group structures and sources of power (such as agendas, chairing a meeting, leadership, etc.). Instead, open, agenda-less groups with no particular person dictating or steering the group are favoured. However, for most work (as opposed, say, to therapy groups) roles and associated power strongholds emerge anyway. Freeman (1970) argues that democratic structuring within a group is essential if people are to be equal group participants. Key features of this type of structure are:

- delegation of specific authority to specific people for specific tasks;
- the requirement that all those with authority are responsible to those who selected them;
- distinction of authority amongst as many people as possible;
- rotation of tasks among individuals;
- allocation of tasks along rational, agreed criteria;
- diffusion of information to everyone as frequently as possible;
- equal access to resources needed by the group.

In this way, she argues, whatever structures are developed by different groups will be controlled by, and responsible to, the group. Power within the group will not then become institutionalized.

In terms of what goes on within group discussions, powerlessness can be maintained by lack of knowledge, dominance by other group members in terms of how much and how fast they talk, lack of clarity about the purpose of the meeting, lack of preparation, lack of acceptance by other members, lack of access to resources (such as typing, advocacy, transport, etc.), and lack of contact with the style of speech and specialist terms used.

Feelings of powerlessness can generate alienation and depression, leading to people withdrawing from group membership and feeling bad. Seeman (cited in Plant, 1987) outlines six ways of expressing powerlessness:

- individual powerlessness ('I have no control – others make decisions about me');
- meaninglessness ('What's the point?');
- normlessness or cynicism ('There's no point doing things properly, the only thing that works is breaking the rules');
- cultural alienation ('People – especially me – don't matter any more. The only thing that matters is the budget');
- self-alienation ('I haven't done as well as I should. I'm a failure');
- social isolation ('I feel so lonely, No one wants to listen to or involve me. I'm the odd one out').

It is easy to see how important it is, in the context of legislative exhortations to encourage service user involvement (National Health Service and Community Care Act 1990), to find ways of working with consumers of heath care as equals (Brandon and Brandon, 1987; Hallett, 1987). Perhaps ironically, groups themselves can be a source of empowerment (Gibson, 1979; Mullender and Ward, 1991; Whittaker, 1985). It is partly the process of developing and contributing to the group over time that empowers the members. The same could be said of professionals building teams from scratch or for greater effectiveness.

TEAM DEVELOPMENT

As teams meet over time they move through different stages, each characterized by an emphasis on different team activities. While teams may well progress through each stage as they develop over time, they may re-enter an 'earlier' stage as circumstances change. Thus team development continues so long as the team is working together.

Tuckman (1965) suggests that there are four stages of group (team) development. These are the stages of forming, storming, norming and performing. By the last stage the team is working effectively and cohesively with all members working towards a common aim and using their own strengths to best effect. Tuckman's process of team development emphasizes the interpersonal relationships between team members as determinants of the team's work. Figure 12.2 illustrates the process of effective team development.

Any stage can lead to ineffective teamwork and time should be spent exploring and working on the issues facing teams at this stage.

Team development, then, is concerned with ensuring good working relationships, clarity of purpose and of tasks and appropriate team structures to make this possible. If teams are to work well, members must be able to contribute on the basis of their own skills and strengths.

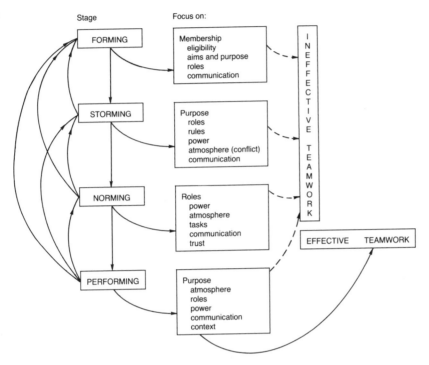

Figure 12.2 Stages of team development and consequences for effective working.

If everyone has the same skills and experience to offer or if they are all expected to carry out the same tasks, the team will not work effectively. Belbin (1981) argues that a balance of different ways of working is needed in effective management teams. He suggests eight 'work types', each with strengths and weaknesses that can be compensated for by their strengths. Table 12.2 summarizes these types.

It can be useful to allocate each team member a 'type' and then share perceptions of each other and identify gaps in the team's strengths. This helps build trust between team members.

MULTIDISCIPLINARY TEAMWORK

The idea of people having their own strengths which they bring to work teams is especially important in multidisciplinary teams and may take some exploration as the team begins to work together, the nature of the work changes or new people join the team.

Whenever a group of people form a team it takes some time (the forming and storming stages) before they fully identify with the team

Table 12.2 Work 'types' and team participation (adapted from Belbin, 1981)

Type	Strengths	Allowable weakness
'Plant' or ideas person	Creative, imaginative, good at solving problems	Head in the clouds, poor at communicating
Resource investigator	Extrovert, enthusiastic, communicative, explores opportunities, networks	Loses interest quickly
Coordinator	Confident, trusting, promotes joint decision making	Not very clever or creative
Monitor–evaluator	Strategic, serious, considers all options, judges accurately	Unable to motivate others
Shaper	Dynamic, extrovert, highly-strung, challenges inertia of ineffectiveness, finds solutions	Short-tempered and easily provoked
Team worker	Sociable, perceptive, accommodating, listens and avoids friction	Indecisive in crises
Implementor	Reliable, disciplined, conservative, efficient, good organizer	Inflexible, slow to respond to new ideas
Completer–finisher	Conscientious, anxious, detects and corrects errors, orderly, perfectionist	Worries about small things, difficulty letting go
Specialist	Single-minded, dedicated	Contributions rather narrow

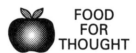

FOOD FOR THOUGHT

What difference does it make to multidisciplinary teams if members blur their roles? Consider this in relation to a) a community mental health team, b) a child abuse case conference and c) the care team for a terminally ill woman with melanoma.

Does a mixture of ages make for more effective work teams?

Where are conflicts likely to arise in multidisciplinary health teams?

What ways are there of building teams whose members assume different values, come from different cultures and include both men and women?

itself. All team members are also members of other groups – such as age, sex, interest, family, cultural groups.

The force of these previous (and often still existing) groups may introduce some potential for conflict into the new team before it even gets started. This is particularly likely for multidisciplinary teams. Multidisciplinary teams are made up of people who already identify to some extent with their different professional groups.

The social psychology of intergroup behaviour has drawn attention to the possibility that intergroup hostility will occur simply as a result of categorizing people into different groups (Brewer and Kramer, 1985; Tajfel, 1982b). So nurses identify as nurses and perceive physiotherapists as belonging to another group, and *vice versa*. As soon as people come together, their differences (due to their other group identifications) can create feelings of superiority and hostility.

Consider, for example, the community mental health team working with elderly people with dementia. The social work members prioritize the autonomy and independence of their clients, whereas the nurses prioritize their wellbeing and safety. When the team is asked by case assessors to contribute to the assessment of a particular elderly woman, who will do it? Will each trust the other to do it properly and with the correct emphasis?

It may well be the case that the two groups of workers can work well together until there is some crisis that polarizes them according to their other group memberships and identity (see Brown, 1988 for a review of these issues).

SUMMARY

This chapter has been concerned with skills of working in and with groups. Specifically, the following issues were raised.

- Whenever three or more people exert mutual influence on each other they are said to be a group.
- A group is an abstraction used to define particular forms of interpersonal behaviour and experience.

- The fluctuations in behaviour within groups is known as group dynamics.
- A useful distinction is to be made between group structures and group processes.
- Channels of communications influence experience in groups.
- Communication patterns in groups depend on group structures.
- The nature of communication within groups affects the satisfaction of group members.
- Boys and men dominate communication in mixed sex groups.
- Task and socio-emotive functions of groups are maintained by patterns of communication.
- The nature of interaction processes within groups can be monitored, analysed and changed.
- During group interaction, group roles concerned with task and socio-emotive functions emerge.
- Understanding the roles played within a group may help us understand the effectiveness of a group.
- Effective leadership changes over time and depends on a number of factors, including clarity of task, relationships between group members and authority.
- Different leadership styles are suitable for different purposes and situations.
- Power in groups may be used constructively or destructively.
- Empowerment through group activity needs careful planning and attention to detail.
- Powerlessness in groups may lead to withdrawal from the group activity.
- Teams are particular forms of groups and go through a number of distinct stages of development.
- The interpersonal relationships between team members determine the efficacy of the team's work.
- Effective teams allow individual members to make different contributions.
- Teams work best with a balance of team members' strengths and weaknesses.
- Intergroup hostility can result from multiple group membership.
- Interprofessional conflict can be understood as a particular form of intergroup hostility.
- A common identity is important in multidisciplinary teams.

SELF-DEVELOPMENT EXERCISES

1. When does a collection of people become a group? Think about a situation at work recently when a previously unconnected group of people began to cohere as a group.

2. Next time you are involved in a group, try to record patterns of communication. Draw the group structure on a piece of paper, marking each person with a letter. When one person talks to another constructively, join them with a solid line. When they talk to each other destructively, join them with a dotted line. Try to do this for the duration of the group discussion. Look at the pattern you now have. Where is the power in the group located? What is the source of the power within the group? Does everyone contribute to the talk equally? If not, what patterns emerge?

3. Watch a group discussion on television. Try to record the discussion in terms of Bales's interaction categories. How easy or difficult did you find this? Why? What differences might there be in trying to describe interaction patterns in a live group of which you are a member? What are the limitations of this type of group process recording?

4. Think of a group that you regularly participate in. What roles do the different members occupy? Are these task or socio-emotive roles? Do the same people play the same roles each time you meet? How easy would it be for regular group members to adopt a completely different role within the group? Why?

5. Think about your own work team. Write a job description for the team leader describing all s/he is to do, and how s/he is to do it, across a number of different work situations.

6. Imagine you have been given some European Community funding to involve people who receive nursing services in planning the service for the future. You have to put a proposal to the EC stating how you will do this. What will you include in your proposal?

7. Plan a team-building day for your own work team. Include an analysis of the team's current stage of development and the extent to which it works effectively. What will you focus on during the team-building day and why? How might you follow this day up in order to ensure effective teamwork?

8. Describe your own work team in terms of Belbin's team roles. If possible, get other team members to do the same. Share your analysis with each other. Are any of the roles missing or duplicated? If so, what are the implications for the effective working of the team and for team development?

CHAPTER 13

Supervision and appraisal

Over the last decade nurses have had to engage with the interpersonal processes of appraisal, performance review and professional supervision (Butterworth and Faugier, 1992). Performance review came about because of changed management arrangements in the Health Service and is generally confined to those eligible for performance-related pay. Appraisal is more widespread and is used in different contexts. It can be a regular opportunity to appraise progress in a job; it can be the term used in remedying deficiencies in how the job is being done; it can be used in exit counselling at times of relocation or redundancy as a result of reorganization; it can be used to refer to the process of examining the nature of a job and the skills required to do it in a grading or re-grading claim. Appraisal may or may not be linked to promotion. Professional supervision, too, has different meanings in different contexts. Many people receiving supervision think of it as being watched over and checked for poor practice: indeed, this view is not unfounded in those situations where supervision is only introduced when a problem has arisen with a particular nurse or job.

Consider, for example, a health visitor working with a family whose children are on the at-risk register. At one case conference the health visitor's work is called into question. She is accused of over-involvement and collusion with the mother. During the case conference her manager assures the other professionals that she will introduce close supervision of the health visitor's work on a regular basis, in order to avoid professional over-involvement. As a result the health visitor feels criticized, unsupported and vulnerable. When she is asked to attend a supervision session she feels resentful and defensive. Soon after she goes off sick and then gets another job in a neighbouring community trust. Here, regular supervision is seen as an essential part of a quality health visiting service. It is included in the job description and training is received during the induction period. Now, the health visitor feels supported, valued and able to admit to professional dilemmas.

THE NATURE OF SUPERVISION

Supervision is generally considered to be a supportive system that enables staff to work more effectively. As Metcalfe and Curtis (1992) say: 'Supervision is where individuals and the organization meet to communicate, resolve respective demands, make decisions, and agree the objectives and tasks that produce a required level of service. Supervision concerns the direction, support and development of the worker, group or team, as they adopt their skills to meet new service demands' (p. vi). Supervision then, can help support staff in day to day activities, and through major change (Kagan, 1992). It can help staff manage their personal resources and their workloads, cope with stress, find more effective ways of coping (Kagan and Child, 1993) and increase their job satisfaction (Cherniss and Egnatios, 1978).

Depending on workers' requirements at any particular point in time, the focus of supervision can be on management, education or support (Kadushin, 1976). In practice, these areas overlap and there are many instances where managerial, supportive and educative consideration intermingle (Hawkins and Shohet, 1989).

DEVELOPMENTAL APPROACH TO SUPERVISION

Not only do workers' needs within supervision change from week to week, they may also change over the course of their career. As they develop as nurses, their needs within supervision change (Hawkins and Shohet, 1989). Schmidt (1973) suggests four levels of worker development.

Stage 1: High anxiety

This stage occurs during the first 3–6 months on the job. Exposure to pressure, upset in patients and relatives, and personal upset may result in confusion. Nurses may be searching for ways to respond to and examine personal feelings towards patients. This stage can be precipitated whenever work becomes emotionally charged.

Stage 2: 'Make it or break it'

Nurses have developed knowledge and skills, giving them confidence in making plans and decisions. They may still experience some anxiety and have limited ability to identify mistakes. This stage can be precipitated by moving to a new job or handling change in existing job.

Stage 3: Skilled assessment and intervention

Nurses are able to identify and analyse errors. Basic knowledge has been incorporated and they are able to identify gaps in their work with patients. Nurses begin to set personal and professional goals. This stage is the beginning of independent practice.

Stage 4: Relative independence

Nurses can identify problems and options and generally can determine most of the agenda for supervision. They may have a good idea of their supervision needs and of what is required to further their professional development.

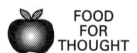

**FOOD
FOR
THOUGHT**

What difficulties are there for experienced staff being supervised by less experienced staff?

Is it easier to supervise same-sex or opposite-sex staff?

How do cultural differences affect the willingness of staff to raise matters of concern with supervisors?

Are different supervisory skills indicated for supervising nurses at different stages?

How easy is it to determine the stage of development a) you or b) others are in?

STYLES OF SUPERVISION

At the heart of supervision are the helping skills of supervisors. Heron (1975) has categorized facilitating or enabling intervention into six groups, as shown below.

These groups represent different ways of helping: they also reflect different styles of supervision. Most of us feel more comfortable using particular styles or actual helping skills. The major styles underpinning

Supervisory intervention skills (after Heron, 1975)

Prescriptive
Give advice, be directive, e.g., 'You need to write a report on that'; 'The next stage is to let the relatives know'

Informative
Be didactic, instruct, perform, e.g., 'You will find the procedures outlined in the operational policy'; 'This is how we deal with residents' money'

Confrontative
Be challenging, give direct feedback, e.g., 'I notice that when you talk about her mother you always smile'; 'You seem to object to the amount of information given to families when their child comes for audiological surgery'

Cathartic
Release tension, enable feelings to be expressed, e.g., 'What is it you'd really like to say to your ward sister?'

Catalytic
Be reflective, encourage self-directed problem solving, e.g., 'Can you say some more about that?'; 'What might happen if you did that?'

Supportive
Be approving, confirming, validating, e.g., 'I can understand how you feel'; 'What you said was really helpful'; 'You handled that in the best way possible'

supervision are teaching, managerial or therapeutic styles (Kurpius, Baker and Thomas, 1977). Although it is possible to merge styles (Boyd, 1978), the skilled supervisor is able to use whichever interventions and style are most appropriate for a particular person or situations. Indeed Heron suggests that all six types of intervention are useful if rooted in concern and care for the person being supervised. They are not useful if used in an unskilled or compulsive way and rooted in lack of awareness (those he refers to as **degenerate interventions**). Nor are they useful if used deliberately maliciously (**perverted intervention**).

Table 13.1 Styles of supervision

	Educative	Managerial	Supportive
View of nurse	Technician	Task achiever	Person
Goals and purposes set by	Profession/work unit/ supervisor	Agency/supervisor/work unit	Profession/nurse/supervisor
Philosophy of supervision	'I can show you how to improve or we can learn together'	'I can pinpoint what you should be doing or what you are doing wrong'	'I can help you clarify who you are as a person and as a nurse'
Supervisor–nurse relationship	Superordinate–subordinate	Superordinate–subordinate	Colleagues
Purpose of supervision	Tasks	Job	Interpersonal relationships
Focus	Professional development, knowledge and skills	Organizational performance, skills (including the remediation of weakness)	Thoughts, feelings and beliefs
Power held by	Supervisor (role)	Supervisor (role)	Shared
Tone of supervision	Positive–neutral	Negative–positive	Positive

Different supervision styles lead to different emphases within supervision and are underpinned by different assumptions. Some of these are illustrated in Table 13.1.

PROACTIVE APPROACH TO SUPERVISION

Supervision is an interpersonal encounter and we should not fall into the trap of assuming that the onus is on supervisors to conduct supervision. To do this leads to a view of supervisees as passive recipients of supervision: they get it or they do not; it is good or it is not. A more proactive approach is to see supervision as a joint responsibility between supervisors and supervisees, each bring their own past experiences, expectations and requirements (Hawkins and Shohet, 1989; Kagan, 1993).

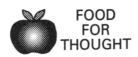

FOOD
FOR
THOUGHT

What are the responsibilities of supervisors in supervision?
What are the responsibilities of supervisees in supervision?
What responsibilities are there to people outside the supervision process?
What expectations might supervisees have of their supervisors in supervision and *vice versa*?
What are the advantages and disadvantages of supervision taking place within line management (i.e., line managers acting as supervisors)?

So we can all ask for or seek supervision if it is not offered. Indeed, part of being self-aware as a worker is to be able to recognize our own need for support and to understand some of our limitations in securing adequate support.

Hawkins and Shohet (1989) suggest a number of blocks that can prevent effective supervision. Similarly, we might have blocks within the process of giving or receiving supervision. These blocks are summarized overleaf.

A proactive approach to supervision requires expectations to be shared and monitored. Both parties have responsibilities to make supervision effective. Hunt (1986) and Proctor (1988) both emphasize the importance of an explicit contract wherein both parties share their

Blocks to getting supervision and to making effective use of supervision

Blocks to getting supervision

Previous experience of supervision: 'A waste of time'; 'Critical and unpleasant'; 'More about my supervisor than me'; 'No one could be as good as she was'

Personal inhibitions: 'I feel uncomfortable when my work is under scrutiny'; 'All I want to do is justify myself'

Difficulties in the supervisory relationship: 'I get worried my supervisor will think badly of me'; 'My difficulty is I think I'm a better worker than he is'; 'I don't trust her'

Organizational blocks: 'My supervisor is also my manager and the person who will write me a reference – how can I be honest about my difficulties?'; 'The rota system doesn't build in supervision'; 'There is nowhere we can go to have a private conversation'

Practical blocks: 'When an important meeting comes up or we're short-staffed, supervision is the first thing to go'; 'We just cannot afford the time for supervision because of the staffing levels'

Culture of the organization or profession: 'Everyone is expected to be able to cope without help;' 'While professional supervision is expected, there is no training available'; 'All they are concerned about is balancing the budget – staff don't matter'

Blocks within supervision

'Blind spots': Well established personal patterns of perception and communication that prevent clarity of thought and expression

'Deaf spots': Personal defences and defensiveness intrude upon honest and open consideration of issues

'Dumb spots': Difficulties expressing empathy with another person

Consider, for example, the psychiatric nurse manager, deeply committed to his hospital-based service, including admissions, observation, long-stay and day wards. He has built up a psychiatric nursing service that works well with psychiatrists. His local purchaser wishes to purchase a service that is not hospital-based and that features multidisciplinary teams. During supervision the process of change is on the agenda. The nurse uses strategies to: a) divert attention from this issue by raising relatively trivial management issues, claiming they are of immediate importance; b) highlight the strengths of the existing service; c) raise issues concerned with the difficulties of working with psychiatrists, occupational therapists and social workers locally. All these strategies can be thought of as games – a) 'You can't catch me and pin me down'; b) 'We are the Champions'; c) 'I have an impossible job as it is'. Unless his supervisor challenges the 'games' he will be able to strengthen his resistance to change. The 'games' may continue out of supervision. For example, he may begin a user-consultation process that supports the 'We are the Champions' game.

expectations, purposes, strategies and outcomes. Figure 13.1 illustrates the components that might be included in a supervision contract.

ENHANCING MOTIVATION AND FEEDBACK

Supervision is more than a conversation: it includes skills of motivating staff and giving feedback. Both the motivation and feedback skills can be incorporated into appraisal and performance reviews as well as supervision.

There are a number of techniques for enhancing motivation and intrinsic interest in the work that nurses do. They are no substitute for good pay and working conditions, but they can make a difference to the quality of work done by nurses. Techniques for motivating staff are summarized overleaf.

While these techniques are geared to enhancing motivation, they are also salient features of good people-management. In the course of encouraging positive motivation and supervision more generally, it will be necessary to give feedback on performance (and to get and receive it). Feedback is a way of helping other people to: a) consider changing their behaviour; b) understand how other people experience them; and c) stay on target and achieve their goals. A useful mnemonic to help remember some key principles of giving good feedback is CORBS (Hawkins and Shohet, 1989). This stands for Clear, Owned, Regular, Balanced and Specific.

Purpose of supervision:

Expectations:
Supervisee   Supervisor

Responsibilities:

                          Supervisor   Supervisee
Identification of issues
Become able to share
Open to feedback
Monitor defensivenes
Evaluate feedback

Agreed 'ground rules':
e.g. Frequency:
       Duration:
       Role of case discussion:
       Role of preparation:
       Confidentiality

Review:
       Frequency
       Nature

Evaluation:
       e.g. Supervisor style
       Content of sessions
       'Fit' with expectations
       Effect on motivation
       Effectiveness at work

Figure 13.1   Components of a contract for supervision.

Techniques for motivating staff at work

Use of appropriate reinforcement
- as close to actual behaviour as possible
- of value to individual nurses
- keep it realistic – too much is as bad as none at all
- balance short-term and long-term incentives

Set up situations when people can be successful
- give opportunities to experience success
- tailor these situations to interests and skills of individual nurses
- recognize individual accomplishment
- point out improvements in performance, no matter how small

Provide flexibility and choice
- wherever possible, allow nurses to make decisions on their own
- enable nurses to have some say over decisions that affect them

Provide support when needed
- nurses should be encouraged to ask for support and assistance
- asking for support should be seen as a sign of strength

Show interest in and knowledge of individual people
- make nurses feel important and personally significant
- get to know each person separately, including their outside interests, family, etc.

Show confidence in staff
- confidence leads to positive performance
- nurses who are expected to do well will do so

Ensure expectations are clear
- clear expectations reduce frustration
- nurses can only monitor their effectiveness if they know what is expected

Encourage workers to set their own goals
- nurses are the best judges of their own capabilities and limitations

Assign work that fits workers' interest and skills
- nurses should be encouraged to identify their professional development needs and to follow these through

Individualize supervision
- different people benefit from different supervisory styles
- some people need closer supervision than others
- provide minimum supervision for optimum performance
- agree individual contracts for supervision

Establish a climate of trust and open communication
- encourage participation from all team members
- whenever possible, the threat of rules and discipline should be discouraged
- attempt to remove obstacles to individual people's effective performance
- listen and deal effectively with staff complaints
- criticize behaviour, not people

Demonstrate own motivation through behaviour and attitude
- be motivated and energetic
- demonstrate positive thinking
- model appropriate behaviour

Clear: What feedback do you want to store and why? Try to reduce ambiguity.

Owned: Feedback is your view – not a general truth. Try to stick to the first person – 'I think you are . . .' not 'You are . . .'.

Regular: Regular feedback is the most useful and avoids the build-up of grievances. Give feedback as near to the event as possible.

Balanced: Try to balance positive and negative feedback over time.

Specific: Try to give specific information in feedback that the person can take or leave. Generalized feedback (e.g., 'You have a poor attitude') does not help the worker do things differently in the future.

The giving and receiving of feedback is similar to the skills of assertiveness. As with assertiveness, we do not have to be passive recipients of feedback. Hawkins and Shohet (1989) suggest a number of ways we can be active in receiving feedback.

- If feedback is not given appropriately, request that it be more clear, balanced, owned, regular and specific.
- Listen to the feedback all the way through without judging it – this avoids defensive responses.
- Try not to explain defensively why things were done as they were, nor explain away positive feedback. Listen to how the other person experiences you and say 'Thank you'.
- Ask for feedback you are not given but would like to hear.

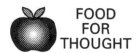

FOOD
FOR
THOUGHT

What are the difficulties of giving and receiving a) positive and b) negative feedback?

When does negative feedback become criticism?

Why do staff lose motivation? Does this vary with experience?

How easy is it for loss of motivation to go unnoticed in a) hospital and b) community settings? Why?

How do feedback skills link with skills of assertiveness and counselling?

In what circumstances would you consider nurses' loss of motivation to be a good thing?

How can you give feedback to someone who does not want to receive it?

Feedback and techniques of motivating staff all involve some negotiation between supervisor and supervisee about each other's perceptions and experiences. If supervision is to be helpful over time it can be a good idea to encourage nurses to set their own objectives and to identify strategies for achieving them.

PERSONAL OBJECTIVES FOR CHANGE

There are several purposes in setting personal learning objectives. Doing so:

- tells us which direction we are going in and whence we have come;
- gives us an indication of change over time;
- specifies what is to be achieved and thereby what is needed to reach this point;
- enables development strategies to be anticipated and communicated to others;
- acts as a motivator and a focus of our work and personal development;
- enables resources to be attracted;
- aids planning.

Personal objectives can be at any level – they might focus on tasks, organizational goals, service user outcomes, personal skills, and so on – but they all imply change and development at an individual level. Supervision, appraisal and performance reviews can all help nurses identify personal objectives. Another useful mnemonic can be applied to objective setting, giving reminders of key features. This is SPIRO (Specificity, Performance, Involvement, Realism, Observability).

Specificity: setting out exactly what is to be accomplished;

Performance: clarifying what behaviours are implied;

Involvement: agreeing who is going to do what;

Realism: being honest about whether it can be done;

Observability: ensuring that a difference in achievement can be seen and assessed by others.

When we set personal development objectives, we may well set several and then have to choose between them. Even at a personal level, this decision making must take several things into account if the objectives stand any chance of being achieved. The social problem-solving process discussed earlier is a useful one. However, when setting personal development objectives, it might be premature to suggest that there is already an identified problem. Indeed, the setting of objectives might partly be creating a problem or goal to be achieved. The GRASP (Getting Results and Solving Problems) process extends the problem-solving process in one important way. It takes as a starting point not the problem *per se*, but a vision of what we wish to achieve. A cyclical process is proposed, as illustrated in Figure 13.2.

When we are selecting between objectives for priority, or between

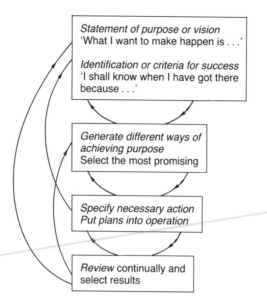

Figure 13.2 Effective problem solving: GRASP (adapted from Comino Foundation Model for Effective Problem Solving, King Alfred's College, Winchester).

strategies for achieving them we need to know criteria along which different objectives or strategies can be compared. Once we compare them, it might be obvious which to pursue first. Figure 13.3 gives an example of one way to compare objectives in terms of who will benefit, what will benefit, and likely timescale.

The role of supervision, appraisal or performance review is to support individual nurses in setting their development objectives and identifying strategies for achieving them. In many ways this process is similar to that of organizational change outlined by Lewin (1951). In his influential text, Lewin proposed a sequence of unfreezing–change–refreezing to summarize the process.

Unfreezing: A person must experience some kind of disequilibrium in the *status quo* of their 'life space'. Once this tension is recognized, a need for change or development is established.

Change: The person tests the proposed changes in real life situations, especially those implying new behaviours or attitudes.

Refreezing: Those new behaviours or attitudes that are more productive are reinforced and internalized. They now contribute to a state of equilibrium in the 'life field'.

This development process forms the basis of experiential learning. One way to view supervision, appraisal and performance review is that they all encourage experiential learning in the nurses giving and receiving supervision, appraisal or review.

Personal Development Objective
(tick those that apply or score 1–5)

objective:	1	2	3	4	5	etc.
Who will benefit most? Myself My colleagues My manager My patients My work . . etc. *What will benefit most?* Quality of my nursing Relationships with colleagues My career Organizational Change . . etc. *What timescale is likely?* Immediate Weeks Months Years . . etc.						

Figure 13.3 Comparisons of personal learning objectives in terms of their likely impact.

APPRAISAL AND PERFORMANCE REVIEW

While many of the issues discussed above in relation to supervision are also relevant in appraisal and performance review, the latter two situations are, perhaps, more focused in terms of how they fit within organizational and management systems. Scott and Rochester (1984) suggest a number of 'rules' for appraisal that should fit any system. These are outlined overleaf.

Appraisal and performance review both incorporate the setting of individual targets linked to action plans. Action plans are a means whereby we can begin to identify ways of achieving goals or targets and as such form part of the social problem-solving process. The key to successful action plans is specificity. They are most useful if they specify the goals, the strategies, method of implementing the strategy, the time scale and precisely how progress will be monitored. There are lots of similar procedures within nursing practice, including implemen-

Key issues for effective appraisal

- The first purpose of appraisal is to improve a person's performance in the present job
- A second purpose is to see what potential she or he might have for other jobs in the organization
- The manager doing the appraisal should be the immediate boss of the person appraised
- Discussion of performance should be based on objective standards
- Both the person and the appraiser need to prepare for the interview
- Criticism does not improve anyone's abilities
- The appraiser needs to listen
- The aim is to work out a plan
- Helping anyone to do a job better is a day-to-day responsibility for her/his manager
- Pay is not a subject for discussion during appraisals

tation of the nursing process, individual care plans and care management (Kagan, 1990)

Supervision, appraisal and performance review are all examples of social problem solving. They are complex interpersonal situations building on the fundamental interpersonal processes of speech, non-verbal behaviour and social perception via active listening and facilitation skills. Contemporary interest in quality services and quality of nursing care, coupled with specifications of nursing standards via contracting, has highlighted the essential roles appraisal and performance review play in maintaining effective nursing practice (Burton, 1992; Kagan, 1992; Kagan and Child, 1993).

SUMMARY

This chapter has been concerned with supervision, appraisal and performance review. Specifically, the following issues were raised.

- Supervision, appraisal and performance review differ in terms of their organizational functions.

- Supervision is a supportive system that enables staff to work more effectively, manage their personal resources and workloads and increase their job satisfaction.
- The focus of supervision may be on managerial, supportive or educational issues.
- Individual nurses' supervision needs develop over time.
- Different stages of worker development are characterized by different staff concerns.
- Supervisors may use different styles of supervision with different people at different times.
- Different supervisory intervention skills achieve different outcomes.
- Some intervention strategies are unhelpful.
- A proactive approach to supervision recognizes the contribution made to the process by both supervisor and supervisee.
- Nurses' previous experiences, personal inhibitions or interpersonal difficulties may create blocks to seeking supervision and making constructive use of supervision.
- There may be organizational or cultural blocks to effective supervision.
- Those involved in supervision may have personal blocks within the supervision process.
- Nurses sometimes play games in supervision.
- Monitoring and evaluating the supervision process contributes to open and constructive supervision.
- Supervision contracts can clarify both expectations and procedures of supervision.
- Supervision can play an important part in motivating staff if techniques are used skilfully.
- Constructive feedback is the key to effective supervision, and should be clear, owned, regular, balanced and specific.
- Giving and receiving feedback are skills closely allied to assertive skills.
- Personal objectives for change can be identified within supervision.
- Prioritizing and choosing between personal objectives for change involves a decision-making process that can be aided by supervision.
- Personal change *via* supervision is similar to processes of organizational change.
- Supervision, appraisal and performance review all encourage experiential learning.
- Appraisal and performance review are more closely tied in with organizational priorities.
- Action planning is a key feature of appraisal and performance review.
- Supervision, appraisal and performance review are all thought to contribute to the delivery of quality services.

SELF-DEVELOPMENT EXERCISES

1. Think about your own work setting. If you have supervision, what is its purpose? Think of a time you received good supervision (it may not be in the current job). What made it good? What benefits did a) you and b) your organization derive from it?

2. Draw up a proactive supervision contract that would be helpful to you in your work. If possible, do this with someone who is in a position to give you supervision. In your contract, take account of the developmental stage you are at currently. How will you monitor the effectiveness of the supervision?

3. With a friend or a colleague, discuss any problem s/he has. Your task is to be as helpful as possible. Discuss the strategies for helping you used and try to decide which style of helping (teaching, managerial or therapeutic) you adopted. It is probable that you used aspects of all three: try to decide which style was given emphasis. How easy would you find it to adopt a completely different style?

4. What blocks to effective supervision are there in a) your organization, b) you yourself and c) your supervisor? Where do these blocks come from and how might they be overcome?

5. Try to give a colleague some positive feedback about some aspect of her/his work (this does not have to be in the context of supervision). How easy was it to follow the CORBS mnemonic? What makes it difficult? Think how you react to positive feedback from colleagues. Does the impact of the feedback depend on who it is that gives it? Why/why not?

6. Imagine you are in a position to influence the staff in your workplace. What you say, they will do. Devise a poster instructing all your colleagues about the best way to motivate their colleagues. What made you include what you have done?

7. With some colleagues, design a coat of arms for your work team that captures all the best aspects of working where you work, doing the job you do.

8. Draw up a personal action plan, specifying your own objectives for the next year. Outline how you will achieve the objectives and clarify what it would take from the organization to help you achieve them. Try to put your plan into practice.

CHAPTER 14

Handling pressure

There are many different kinds of pressures in nursing that affect different people in different ways. Some people thrive in ever-changing, demanding and challenging situations; others do not. Some people thrive in stable, undemanding and repetitive situations; others do not. Some people thrive in unpredictable and variable situations; others do not. Some people prefer to work alone for long periods of time and others prefer the constant company of colleagues. Nursing can be all of these situations.

Some jobs may reflect one type of situation more than others and some jobs will change over time. All of this means it is a very complex task to describe the nature of pressure in nursing and to predict how different nurses will react to it. How nurses react to pressure and what else is going on in their lives outside work will influence whether their responses are positive or negative. Negative pressure is often referred to as **stress** and may lead to inability to cope with work or a breakdown in relationships at work. Thus the handling of pressure is closely linked to professional interpersonal skills. In terms of our model of interpersonal skill, recognizing and handling stress touches on all the different component parts of interpersonal skill.

THE NATURE OF STRESS

Stress can be examined at both psychological and physiological levels. In reality, physiological and psychological aspects of stress are inter-related (Burchfield, 1985; Weinberger, Hiner and Tierney, 1987).

Psychological perspectives on stress

Discussions of the nature of stress often confuse stress as a precursor (or stimulus) of other events, stress as the experience of events and stress as a reaction (or response) to events (Kasl and Cooper, 1987; Milne and Watkins, 1986). Harvey (1989) suggests that one way of resolving this confusion is to distinguish between **stressors** (the events perceived by a person as stressful), **stress** (the subjective experience)

Consider, for example, the night sister who likes working on her own. The orthopaedic wards she works on are generally quiet at night. However staffing shortages mean she has to cover two acute medical wards too. These are busy with admissions, disturbances and sometimes death at night. The sister will react differently to this increased pressure from another sister who enjoys handling emergencies and coordinating interprofessional teams. Similarly, a nurse supporting people with mental health difficulties in the community who enjoys working closely with others and benefits from being able to discuss issues during the course of the day will experience pressure in her isolated work.

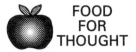

FOOD FOR THOUGHT

Why is it that people react differently to different situations?

How do we learn to see some things as stressful and other things as not stressful?

How can we 'fit' people to jobs appropriate to their skills, qualifications and interests?

What bodily sensations go along with a) feelings of pressure and b) feelings of being unable to cope?

Why do some people experience migraines or get colds immediately following periods of high pressure?

How important is a) the job, b) the home and c) the person in contributing to stress on nurses?

and **stress responses** (the behaviour and reactions to stressors that occur). Thus, in order to experience stress or show stress responses, a person has to both perceive and label the stressors as such. Events are not, therefore, inherently stressful and do not necessarily lead to stress responses. As Harvey says: 'The actual experience and responses made will depend on the context in which the event is experienced ...

"stress" is seen as a dynamic interactional process rather than a single event or set of responses' (Harvey, 1989, p. 25).

Cox (1978) also highlighted the importance of the ways different demands are perceived. He emphasized the importance of the way people perceive their own abilities to meet demands placed upon them. Both 'underload' and 'overload' of demands may be stressful. Thus nurses who perceive themselves to be more highly qualified and skilled than the job they are doing may experience stress. Similarly, nurses who perceive themselves to be under-qualified or to lack the skills or temperament for the specific job may experience stress.

The experience of stress, then, arises from a perceived mismatch between demands on nurses and their ability to cope with those demands. However, the experience of stress and the effectiveness of coping are affected by both the amount of control or power people can exert in coping and the nature and family of supports they receive from others (Cohen and McKay, 1984).

Physiological perspectives on stress

The above discussion emphasizes the psychological aspects of stress. While many of the psychological consequences of stress (such as lack of ambition, interpersonal conflict, depression, low morale, anxiety, possibly burnout) are well known, there can also be physical consequences of stress, leading to illness (Kasl and Cooper, 1987; Elliott and Eisdorfer, 1982). Long before psychological accounts of stress were developed, physiological responses to stress were described. In 1956 Selye described the 'stress response' or general adaptation syndrome (GAS). GAS is the bodily reaction to threats of damage to bodily systems. Selye (1980) suggested that the body responds in a relatively constant way regardless of the type of stressor, while the degree of response varies with the extent of demand for adjustment. Three stages to GAS were identified; alarm, resistance and exhaustion, with various physiological changes at each stage (see Kaplan, Sallis and Patterson, 1993 or Niven, 1989 for further discussion) that affect the endocrine, cardiovascular and immune systems. It is because of the physiological changes that occur that stress is linked to coronary heart disease and some failures of the immune system, in terms either of reducing resistance to mild viral infections or increasing susceptibility to some cancers.

Blood or urine tests are required to monitor the physiological aspects of stress. Psychological aspects of stress can be monitored by what people say and do or by their responses to questionnaires asking them about the nature of their work, reactions and life experiences (Cohen, 1988; Holmes and Rahé, 1967; Kanner *et al.*, 1981; Kasl, 1983; Maddi and Kobasa, 1984; Price, 1982).

INTERPERSONAL SKILLS AND STRESS

The relevance of stress for the professional interpersonal skills of nurses is twofold. Firstly, patients and relatives may experience stress and exhibit stress responses. Nurses may themselves be stressors, or be at the receiving end of patients' or relatives' stress responses. Good nursing care will include the ability to detect when patients and relatives experience stress and either help reduce the stressors or help the patients and relatives cope more effectively.

Secondly, nurses may themselves experience stress and exhibit stress reactions. Their coping mechanisms, ability to monitor their own stress levels and reduce stressors on themselves and their colleagues will all require interpersonal skill.

The rest of this chapter will concentrate on stress at work for nurses, rather than stress for patients and relatives, although discussion of stress in health and illness more generally can be found elsewhere (Bailey and Clarke, 1989).

Copp (1988), after reviewing the literature on stress in nursing, emphasizes the point that nurses cannot expect to avoid demanding stimuli in their jobs. Nevertheless, more could be done to ensure more effective coping, better person–job fit, greater recognition of stressors and social support, the inclusion of stress management in nurse education and the development of greater insight and self-awareness throughout the profession (Bailey and Clarke, 1989; Bond, 1986; Claus and Bailey, 1980; Hawkins, 1987; Parkes, 1980; Smith, 1992).

STRESSORS IN NURSING

Ehrenfeld and Cheifetz (1990) identified three sources of stress for cardiac nurses: relations with staff, relations with patients' families and work-related issues such as overload or inadequate resources.

Sources of pressure for nurses working in community settings went beyond this. Kagan and Child (1993) highlighted aspects of the job, the role, the supports, the work context and the individual nurses themselves that either reduced or increased pressure on staff. These differences are outlined in Table 14.1.

In addition to these factors, Kagan and Child drew attention to the interface between home and work. Family problems, dual career households, life or domestic crises all have the potential to increase pressure at work (Lewis and Cooper, 1989; Cohen, 1988; Brown and Harris, 1989).

Life events

Life events can add to stress for nurses. It might be that a nurse is managing high levels of pressure at work and caring for some very

Table 14.1 Sources of increased or reduced pressure on staff working in community settings (reproduced by kind permission of the North Western Training and Development Team)

	Job	Role	Supports	Context	Person
What is helpful or reduces pressure?	Flexible hours; variety; appropriate recruitment and selection; good fit between worker and job	Have a say; control over working environment; good values and philosophy; shared, clearly defined roles and tasks	Peer contact; supportive colleagues; good working relationships; regular and constructive supervisors who help staff find their own solutions to stress management; appropriate induction and continuing training; management interest; personal back-up services; valued by colleagues and given feedback; emergency back-up; staff counselling	Good and regular communications; opportunities to exercise control over working environment; vigilance for stress	Commitment, enthusiasm and motivation; good interpersonal skills; personal insight; flexibility; effective coping strategies; good time management; feeling in control; constructive outlook; supportive contacts

Table 14.1 Continued

	Job	Role	Supports	Context	Person
What is unhelpful or increases pressure?	Long shifts; paperwork; no contact with others; clients with challenging, aggressive or dangerous behaviour; parental over-involvement; job descriptions inaccurate; boredom; long shifts and lack of rotation between most demanding clients	Undermined in decision making; have to say no because of lack of resources; powerlessness; compromise; lack of clarity about who the client is; no one to share with or to delegate to	Low morale of colleagues; little opportunity for informal contact; required to work in excess of grade; irrelevant induction training; no back-up services and atmosphere of reluctance to admit to personal difficulties; unpredictable emergency back-up	Uncertain future; no consultation; little delegation; budgetary constraints	Feeling of frustration; over-responsibility; clash with colleagues; domestic/personal crises; beliefs that all staff should cope all of the time; no support at work or at home

demanding patients and is coping well. However, a major change in her life occurs which just tips the balance and means she can no longer cope with things at work.

Consider, for example, the community nurse who is working in an inner-city area. His work is full of minor frustrations (such as lifts not working in high-rise flats, traffic jams and diversions, patients not keeping appointments, and so on). The work itself is emotionally demanding as he cares for a large number of people who have been discharged from hospital with terminal illnesses and who are poor. Some of the relatives of his patients are involved with drugs. He has had his car broken into and on one occasion found razor blades attached to the underside of his handbrake. Recently he was assaulted when leaving his car to visit a patient. He is showing signs of pressure, becoming irritable with colleagues. Nevertheless, he is thought to be managing well and it has not occurred to his manager that he should receive supervision. It is only when his confused elderly mother-in-law comes to stay with his family that he begins to take time off work for minor illnesses. He becomes more irritable and starts to make mistakes in record keeping.

This example illustrates how people can continue to cope with considerable pressure until circumstances (in this example, domestic) change to just tip the balance away from coping.

While the concept of life events is subject to some criticism (Kasl, 1983) they are often perceived by people to be of importance, although the meaning attached to different life events determines whether or not they are stressful. In general, young people experience a greater number of life events than older people and women tend to accumulate more life changes than men (Goldberg and Comstock, 1980). Of course younger people and women may perceive life events in particular ways that mean they either are or are not stressful.

Life events are usually fairly major occurrences (close bereavements, changing jobs, moving house, and so on). Many of the events that people experience are more minor and may even give them a positive boost. Kanner *et al.* (1981) proposed that minor hassles such as losing one's keys, telephones not working, reports being delayed, and so on contribute to stress. However, these irritants can be counterbalanced by uplifts, such as getting on well with colleagues, completing a piece of work, feeling fit, and so on.

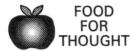 FOOD
FOR
THOUGHT

How does the experience of life events such as moving house, changing jobs, unemployment, coping with illness of a family member, vary with a) age, b) sex and c) cultural background?

What euphemisms for coping are there (e.g., 'tower of strength')? How do these affect our experiences of coping and lack of coping?

How important are daily hassles in pressurizing nurses at work?

Why is change stressful? What makes it less so?

What scope is there for nurses of different grades to retain control over change at work?

Are any of the interpersonal strategies nurses use to cope with the emotional demands of the job beneficial? Which ones and how?

Transitions such as being allocated to a new locality in the community, working with a new team of people or moving to a different specialty, constitute particular kinds of life event requiring adjustment over time (Adams, Hayes and Hopson, 1976; Felner, Farber and Primavera, 1985). Transitions involve meeting the demands of previously unfamiliar people, tasks and situations. They also require some adjustment. However, in the long run, transitions can often be positive.

Organizational change contributes to pressure. In recent years nursing, along with the rest of the health service, has undergone considerable upheaval. Many nurses have been relocated to other posts and care practices have changed. These changes may be seen as transitions, and as such may lead to transition stress, depending how they are perceived. Organizational change rarely takes place without some reallocation or a cut in resources. While this may lead to increased or changing workloads, the aspect about resourcing that leads to most stress is the perception many nurses have of being powerless to influence the course of events. Feelings of lack of control and powerlessness contribute to stress.

Life events and demands at work do not necessarily lead to stress. In the face of many potential stressors some people remain healthy.

Kobasa, Hilker and Maddi (1979) identified two types of people, those who became ill under stress and those who did not. Those who did not had a strong sense of self, believed they were in control, were interested in change, wanted to achieve, showed a capacity for endurance and did not feel threatened by others. Kobasa, Hilker and Maddi introduced the concept of 'hardiness' to describe those least susceptible to stress. Hardiness has been identified as a characteristic that lessens the likelihood that nurses will experience burnout as a result of work stress (McCrane, Lambert and Lambert, 1987). The availability of social support, too, alleviates the negative consequences of potential stressors (Howden and Levison, 1987; Faugier, 1991; Firth *et al.*, 1986; Hiscox, 1991).

Coping

In dealing with the experience of stress, people use different coping mechanisms. Coping can be directed at a) removing stressors, b) the experience of stress and c) the response to stress. Pearlin and Schooler (1978) define coping as things people do to avoid being harmed by life strains. Lazarus and Folkman (1984) provide a more complex definition that takes account of different types of stressors and different experiences of them. For them, coping is made up of behavioural and cognitive activities used to manage (master, tolerate, reduce and minimize) environmental and internal demands – and conflicts among them – which tax or exceed a person's resources. Coping is not a single strategy: different people cope differently with hassles, major life events, perceived over- and underload, and so on.

Some of the earliest explorations of nurses' coping strategies were based on the notion of coping mechanisms as defence mechanisms (Menzies, 1960). They are based on psychoanalytic concepts and assume that coping protects nurses and enables them to work in emotionally demanding and threatening situations. Thus in order to avoid potential emotional overload, nurses may speak and act in particular ways, blocking emotional expression and recognition (Macleod Clark, 1983; Menzies, 1960). From the same perspective, tension-reduction strategies for responding to stress (for example relaxation training, autogenic training, meditation) may be used as coping strategies. It is worth remembering that defensive coping strategies may be adaptive or maladaptive.

Personal characteristics or styles may lead to adaptive or maladaptive coping. A lot has been written and researched about 'Type A' and 'Type B' behaviour patterns and their contributions to stress (Friedman and Rosenman, 1974; Looker and Gregson, 1989). Very briefly, people exhibiting greater amounts of 'Type A' behaviour would be more likely to display competitiveness, hostility, intense job involvement, impatience and time-urgency. People who exhibit 'Type A' behaviour may create stress by over-reacting to every potential stressor and are thus in a constant state of physical arousal. In many nursing situations, 'Type A' behaviour is explicitly encouraged, with high achievement targets and performance objectives.

'Type B' behaviour patterns are characterized by the opposite behaviours: 'Type B' behaviour is less competitive and more cooperative. People have less intensive job involvement, more patience and are not time-bound. Although 'Type A' and 'Type B' behaviour will vary with different situations, in general people who display 'Type A' behaviour are more prone to stress (and in extreme cases, coronary heart disease). The behaviour patterns can, however, be modified. An effective coping strategy for people prone to 'Type A' behaviour would be to learn to use more 'Type B' behaviours.

Consider, for example, the emphasis on patient or client contact as a major performance indicator in some nursing contexts. A nurse who is expected to increase the number of patients s/he works directly with, irrespective of the nature of the contact, is encouraged to increase turnaround, to decrease time spent with individual patients and to cut the time spent on administrative tasks. This is explicit encouragement of 'Type A' behaviour. If performance on these criteria form the basis of promotion, 'Type A' behaviour is ingrained in the structures of the nursing service. Willingness to work extra hours or to take work home is often thought to reveal showing motivation and commitment to the job, and may therefore be recognized and rewarded as such. It is, again, though, 'Type A' behaviour. Nurses caught up in this way of working may do well to learn to say 'no'; to recognize that they cannot do absolutely everything to very high standards and to pace their work more realistically – in other words to develop 'Type B' behaviour.

Lazarus and Folkman (1984) have proposed a cognitive–phenomenological approach to coping. From this perspective people and their environments are viewed as ongoing transactions, each affecting and being affected by the other. Cognitive appraisal is the process by which an event is evaluated in terms of a) what is at stake in terms of the personal harm that may be caused (primary appraisal) and b) what coping responses are available (secondary appraisal).

To the extent that a person feels harmed, threatened or challenged, she or he will experience stress. Each situation and event is appraised differently and different types of coping are used. Lazarus (1966) suggested that coping could be separated into problem-focused and emotion-focused types of response. Billings and Moos (1981) extended this categorization to include both cognitive and behavioural aspects of problem-focused and emotion-focused coping. Different types of response can be organized as shown below.

Cognitive and behavioural coping responses

Cognitive: emotion-focused
- Try to see positive side
- Try to stand apart from the event
- Pray for guidance

Cognitive: problem-focused
- Consider alternative ways of having problem
- Take one step at a time
- Use past experiences

Behavioural: problem-focused
- Collect information
- Talk with knowledgeable person
- Take some positive action
- Talk with spouse, friend or relative
- Confrontation

Behavioural: emotion-focused
- Seek support
- Physical exercise
- Meditation
- Use of alcohol
- etc.

Ehrenfeld and Cheifetz (1990) draw out the links between behavioural and emotional aspects of different kinds of coping strategies used by nurses. They are, they suggest, interlinked parts of coping strategies and cannot be separated. They identify four modes of coping with stress that highlight the interpersonal nature of most nurses' stressful situations. The coping modes they identify are:

- active coping towards solution;
- diverting responsibility to others;
- passivity;
- activity that is not geared to problem solving.

No one coping strategy is adaptive in all situations, and Steptoe (1991) argues that all coping responses have physiological costs as well as benefits. What is adaptive may well depend on what physiological processes are most adaptive to particular individuals. For example, a person suffering from coronary artery disease needs to avoid strategies which increase sympathetic nervous system activity (for example hard physical exercise), whereas other people may benefit from them.

Dewe (1991) explores the link between primary and secondary appraisal and stressful encounters at work. While it may well be that different coping responses will benefit people differently in different situations there are some indications that the experience of stress at work has both personal and organizational consequences and that features of the work can act as stressors.

Burnout in nursing has received extensive and widespread interest and is thought to be a consequence of maladaptive coping with perceived stress (Maslach 1982; Paine, 1982). Low morale and job dissatisfaction are both causes and consequences of burnout, leading people to become ill and sometimes to leave the profession (Crotty 1987; Dolan 1987; Gaze, 1988; McConnell, 1982). Changes in conditions at work as well as personal coping strategies can help prevent burnout. Table 14.1 outlined some of the features of community nursing that helped reduce pressure on staff.

Vigilance for stress

Vigilance for stress at work is everyone's responsibility and attention should be paid to every aspect of the job to ensure the right person is doing the right job in the right way in the right situation. Kagan and Child (1993) identified a number of work systems that can help and reduce stress linked to the job, the role, available supports and the context of the work. In diagnosing and remedying occupational stress, all the systems outlined in Table 14.2 should be looked at regularly by all involved.

Managers play a key part in ensuring that their workplaces do not put such pressures on staff that they cannot cope with the work. If stressors are so great the service will suffer and patients will not receive good nursing care. A combination of organizational and per-

Table 14.2 Summary of systems that help reduce and/or prevent stress in community residential settings (reproduced by kind permission of the North Western Training and Development Team)

Sources of stress	Job	Role	Supports		Context
			Formal	Informal	
Job design	*	*			*
Recruitment and selection	*	*	*		*
Induction	*	*			
Training	*	*	*		*
Resource allocation	*	*			*
Guidelines and procedures		*			*
Communications		*	*	*	*
Linked services	*	*	*		
Quality assessment		*	*		
Managerial contact with staff		*	*		*
Promotions and career development		*	*		
Supervision		*	*		
Control	*		*		*
Skills review			*		
Feedback			*	*	*
Peer contact		*		*	*
Team meetings			*	*	
Team building			*	*	
Back-up services			*		*
Time	*	*			
Intake	*				
Energy	*				*
Problem solving	*				
Social changes		*		*	*

sonal strategies for handling pressure should be used, as outlined below.

Organizational and personal strategies for handling pressure

Organization   Individual

Management style   *Behavioural change*
- Participation   - Management of intake
- Communication   – healthy eating
- Supervision   – stop smoking

- Facilitation of individual solutions

Specialist management
- Selection
- Job/person fit
- Training
- Job design

Employees
- Occupational health and welfare systems
- Independent counselling and support
- Health promotion

   – reduce alcohol
- Management of energy
  - exercise regularly
  - relax
  - rest

Psychological change
- Time management
  - assertion
  - development of control
  - plan and manage time
  - prioritize
  - plan for the future
- Emotion-focused strategies
  - express and work through emotions
  - reward self for doing things right
- Problem-focused strategies
  - develop skills and knowledge
  - focus on positive achievements
  - ask for help and advice

Social change
- Develop social contacts at home and work
- Discuss with friends calmly and constructively

Organizational strategies may include regular supervision, the availability of personal counselling, training and career development opportunities, good positive and constructive feedback on work practices and emergency back-up and risk management policies. All of these strategies characterize good management practice.

Figure 14.1 summarizes key aspects of stress in nursing.

SUMMARY

This chapter was concerned with the nature and handling of pressure in nursing. Specifically the following points were raised.

- People differ in their responses to pressure.
- Nursing can involve both positive and negative pressure.

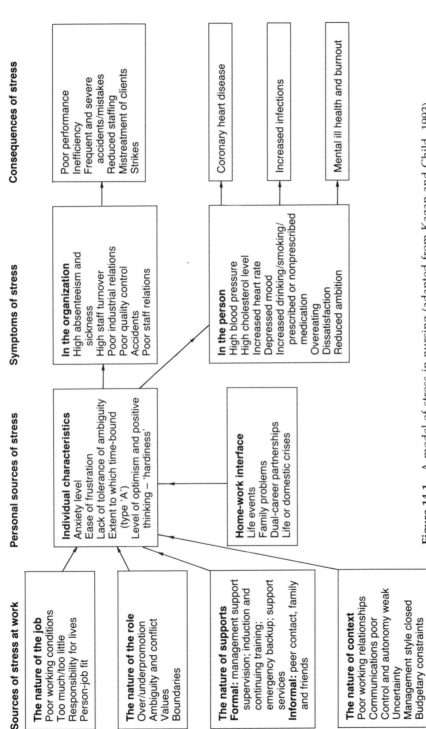

Figure 14.1 A model of stress in nursing (adapted from Kagan and Child, 1993).

- Negative pressure can lead to inability to cope at work.
- Physiological and psychological aspects of stress are inter-related.
- A useful distinction can be made between cause of stress, experience of stress and reactions to stress.
- A mismatch between perceived demands and perceived ability contributes to the experience of stress.
- Stress can have physical consequences linked to the general adaptation syndrome.
- Cardiovascular, endocrine and immune systems can all be affected by stress.
- Stress for nurses can be linked to the nature of the job, the role, the supports, the work context and individual nurses.
- The interface between home and work is important in understanding stress on nurses.
- Life events can increase stress.
- Daily hassles can increase stress.
- Transitions are usually stressful.
- Organizational change creates pressure and often stress.
- 'Hardiness' protects against stress.
- Coping strategies can be directed at removing stressors, experiences of stress or responses to stress.
- Different coping strategies are effective for different people in different situations.
- 'Type A' behaviour leads to stress.
- 'Type A' behaviour may be actively encouraged in nursing.
- Coping strategies may be problem-focused and emotion-focused.
- Occupational stress and burnout can be reduced by changes to the nature, structure and management of work.
- Vigilance for stress is everyone's responsibility.
- Good management practice is an essential part of occupational stress management.

SELF-DEVELOPMENT EXERCISES

1. During one day monitor your own levels of tension. Every hour note the time and what you are doing. Decide how tense you are by giving yourself a tension score (1–3 = low tension; 4–6 = moderate tension; 7–9 = high tension). Try to identify both physical and emotional signs of tension. What fluctuations were there during the day? How typical of an average day was the one you chose? You can do this exercise by thinking back over a day that has nearly passed.
2. How often do you show these physical signs of stress:
   - inability to get to sleep;

- headaches and pains in your head;
- indigestion or sickness;
- unaccountable tiredness or exhaustion;
- fluctuations in what you eat or drink;
- decrease in sexual interest;
- dizziness or shortness of breath;
- muscle twitches;
- pricking sensations in parts of your body;
- unaccountable sweating;
- racing heart?

What do you do about them when you notice them?

3. With colleagues, think about two important problems you face at work. Discuss who is affected, how they are affected, the context in which you work, the impact of the problem on your work. How does the structure of work and the nature of the job contribute to the problem with which you are dealing? Do you have the necessary skills to do the job and deal with the problem?

4. How do you react when you are late for an appointment or for work? How do you react if other colleagues are late for their shift and you have to stay at work a bit longer? Discuss your reactions to lateness with a friend and try to explore whether or not your reactions are reasonable.

5. Design an occupational health education poster that summarizes what all nurses can do about stress at work.

6. Write down all the significant life events you have experienced over the last year. Think about how you managed at times that life events coincided. What recommendations might you give to a friend who is moving house, changing jobs and getting married next Christmas?

7. Identify the ways you relax and wind down from work. Find a new source of relaxation and participate in it regularly for at least six weeks. Monitor the effects it has on your ability to respond to pressure at work.

8. Imagine you are a senior manager who is reorganizing the nursing service in which you work. What would you build into the new service to reduce the likelihood that staff, patients and relatives will suffer ill-effects of stress? How will you check that your systems are keeping stress levels down?

CHAPTER 15

Constraints on using effective interpersonal skills

The effective use of interpersonal skills depends to a large extent on the context in which they are deployed. Those skills effective in one situation may not be so effective in another. However interpersonally skilled we are we may find that our relationships are constrained by factors outside our control. A nurse who is trying to talk to a deaf patient in a noisy crowded room in an understaffed facility where the onus is on physical rather than patient-centred care may well find that her/his efforts are in vain. In this example, the nurse is coming up against factors relating to the patient (deafness), the physical setting (noise, crowding), priorities and funding of health care (understaffing), the organization (physical care emphasis) and possibly her/himself (frustration). In order to try to overcome some of these factors, the nurse must, first of all, learn to recognize them. Even then, though, there will be some factors (such as policy relating to health funding) that s/he will not be able to do anything about. Nurses' recognition of these factors, however, may help them evaluate their own inter-personal skills realistically. The questions we should ask are: 'To what extent do features of the context put realistic constraints on my ability to use interpersonal skills effectively?' and 'To what extent can I adjust my own interpersonal skills in order to make them more effective?'

In this chapter we will look at the context of nursing and explore the range of constraints that surrounded nurses' use of interpersonal skills. These are summarized in Figure 15.1.

We will examine the personal, social and environmental features as well as some of the wider cultural aspects of nursing, with a view to gaining some insight into the extent to which we can deploy effective interpersonal skills as nurses.

PERSONAL CONSTRAINTS

Until fairly recently nurses were not expected to 'get involved' with their patients. It was considered 'professional' to remain detached and

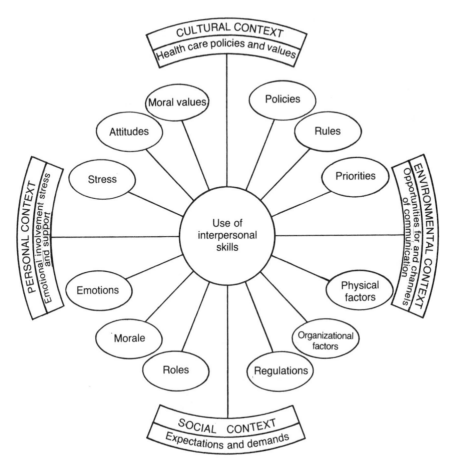

Figure 15.1 Constraints on the effective use of interpersonal skill (from Kagan, Evans and Kay, 1986).

any personal involvement was a breach of professional etiquette. With an emphasis on the interpersonal aspects of nursing, this situation is changing. Nurses are now expected to 'get involved' with their patients in order to best assess their needs and plan and deliver total patient care. This change of emphasis puts enormous pressure on nurses (Llewellyn, 1984, 1989), and the role of the 'self' and self-awareness is central.

Although nurses are expected to get involved with their patients they are not expected to experience the range of emotions that they might experience in other relationships. They are not expected to feel angry, hurt, guilty, hostile, afraid, loving, and so on. And yet of course they do. If we feel unable to gain some control over events we are in danger of experiencing stress (Lazarus and Folkman, 1984). Too much stress can lead to illness (physical and psychological – indigestion, headaches, depression/anxiety), low morale and lack of job satisfaction, all of which, in turn, can lead to nurses giving up their jobs in favour of an occupation that does not exact such a high personal price (Marshall, 1980; Sutherland and Cooper, 1990).

Development of relationships

The implementation of the nursing process, team nursing, primary nursing and the adoption of an interpersonal approach to nursing all put pressure on the individual nurse to form good, warm and often therapeutic relationships with patients (Wright, 1991). That is, in itself, a strange thing to do. In the course of our everyday lives we form relationships out of choice and over a long period of time, rather than because of our role and in a contracted period of time (Marshfield, 1985).

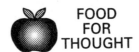

FOOD
FOR
THOUGHT

How much choice is there in forming relationships with a) patients, b) colleagues and c) close friends?

How similar are nurses' relationships with patients to their other personal relationships? How do they differ?

Are relationships with patients two-way?

In what ways do different nursing situations influence the development of nurse–patient relationships?

What kinds of activity can you take part in with a) patients, b) colleagues and c) close friends?

How does the sex, age and cultural background of patients affect nurses' relationships with them?

Relationships with patients do not fit easily into a pattern with which we are familiar in other walks of life. They are distinct and different. Nurses are expected to do intimate, personal things to patients, to share intimate, personal activities with them and to discuss intimate, personal issues with them but at the same time to reveal little that is intimate or personal about themselves. Most relationships elsewhere have an element of reciprocity (sharing) in them. Of course it can be argued that nurses have role relationships and not personal relationships with patients and it is this that distinguishes them (we will consider some of the implications of this later in the chapter). Nevertheless, nurses do get embroiled in the intimate lives of the patients and the consequent drain on their emotional energy may have direct repercussions for patient care (Gow, 1982).

In addition to this, the very existence of particular emotional states (hostility, fear, anger, frustration, etc.) can distort the use of interpersonal skills at all levels (what is said, how it is said, how things are perceived, what courses of action are decided upon, etc.).

Personal support systems

One way in which the stressful effects of the emotional involvement nurses experience can be reduced is by setting up personal support systems (Bailey and Clarke, 1989; Vaughan and Pillmoor, 1989). For some people, personal support is built into the job. Many psychiatric nurses, for example, have frequent case conferences or 'supervision' sessions at which they can vent their feelings about their work, themselves and the people in their care. For others, interpersonal networks are built up wherein groups of nurses often discuss their work and their involvement in it. Others, though, have no opportunity to air their feelings. Family and friends do not like them continually 'talking shop' and colleagues all seem to give the appearance of 'coping'. These are the nurses who are liable to experience the unpleasant effects of stress.

Nursing will always involve a high emotional commitment. However, there is no reason why nurses' emotions should necessarily intrude upon their everyday activities and distort their interpersonal skills. Self-awareness is the first step to being able to overcome the constraints that emotions and personal involvement place on effective interpersonal skills use, and the building of appropriate support systems is the next one. The training of nurses can play a key part in helping nurses find adaptive ways of managing the emotional side of nursing without detriment to interpersonal skill (Smith, 1992). Ideally, we should reach a stage where nurses are able to use 'self' in a therapeutic way, but this will require time and practice in self-exploration and an acknowledgement from the nursing profession at all levels that nurses need and must have personal support at work.

SOCIAL CONSTRAINTS

Social aspects of the nursing context refer to the actual people involved in a particular nursing activity. It makes no sense to talk of nurses' interpersonal skills in isolation from other people. Nurses have inter-action partners, be they patients, colleagues, other health workers or relatives and they all constitute the **interaction context**.

Sutherland and Cooper (1990) draw attention to the occupational role filled by nurses, which is at a boundary. Nurses act between other departments or sections of the health service and between the health service and general public. Such boundary roles are inherently stressful and subject to high role conflict.

ROLES

All these people have roles and associated responsibilities: we have explored the concept of role and its implications for interpersonal skills in Chapter 6. When different people are present in a nursing setting, though, the situation itself may be redefined and this in turn will dictate or prohibit particular repertoires of interpersonal skill. In a hospital ward, for example, different people enter at different times during the day, radically changing the situation for everyone con-cerned, affecting both the way it is perceived and the behaviours that are expected. When the consultant's team enters the ward, nurses (and patients) act differently from when the visitors arrive. It is not the people themselves that have made the difference but their under-standing of the roles they occupy.

We have seen above that nurses might behave differently in their role of nurse. Patients, too, may behave in unpredictable ways that bear little resemblance to their general social behaviour outside the patient role (Wilmott, 1989). Patients are ill. Their illnesses may be distressing, painful, distorting of senses such as sight, hearing, touch or even consciousness. Thus patients, too, might experience increased emotion and distress, which may in turn distort their interactions. It is sometimes suggested that patients are encouraged by health personnel to conform to the 'good' sick role. They are allowed to abdicate their normal social responsibilities and are exempted from responsibility for their conditions, but at the same time are expected to co-operate in order to get well. The 'bad' patients are the uncooperative, questioning people who appear to lack the will to get better. Generally nurses dislike grumbling, complaining, questioning and demanding patients, and liking affects the use of interpersonal skills (Roberts,1984). The ability to overcome factors such as this may distinguish the inter-personal skills of the professional from those of the lay person (Barber, 1989).

Other social factors that may affect interactions include whether or not all the people in a particular situation are of the same age, sex, ethnic background and so on. The relative importance of these factors is difficult to predict and will relate to everyone's past experience, stereotypes and prejudices.

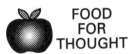

FOOD FOR THOUGHT

How does 'liking' affect interpersonal relationships between nurses and patients?

To what extent do nurses 'overcompensate' when they dislike patients? What effect does this have?

What effect does the way nurses react to irritating patients have on their nursing care?

Are some kinds of patients more demanding than others (e.g., medical/surgical; older/younger; male/female)?

What happens if patients particularly like or dislike individual nurses?

Regulations

In most nursing contexts there are regulations that tell people who occupy different roles how to behave or what to do. These regulations may be clearly stated (explicit) or assumed (implicit). We have considered social rules elsewhere (Chapter 6) but it is useful to think further of how the regulations may constrain the effective deployment of interpersonal skills by nurses.

Consider, for example, a regulation that there should be two community nurses to lift bedridden patients. Staffing levels are such that this is rarely possible. As a consequence, either fewer visits – and thereby fewer chances to talk – are made, or the presence of both nurses on a visit means that intimate conversation is difficult. Similarly, a less formal regulation about the average number of 'client contacts' to be made by community nurses may mean that time spent with any one patient is limited, and the chances to talk intimately reduced. In what circumstances, then, are such disabling regulations to be ignored?

Regulations of the sort mentioned above are closely tied to the organizational context of nursing.

Organizational factors

Organizational factors are those that relate to the ways that nursing activities are structured, and these can constrain nurses' freedom to use their interpersonal skills as they would like to (Faulkner, 1985). In hospitals, the ways in which wards are organized may curtail the opportunities for talking with patients (Burton, 1980; Cullen *et al.*, 1983; Kagan and Burton, 1982). For example, nurses may spend a great deal of time filling in the Kardex system, completing their Korner statistics, or on the phone to other departments. In the community, too, the requirements of administration, the writing of letters, making phone calls, and so on may take up some considerable time (Kagan, 1982). These are the kinds of daily hassles that can contribute to occupational stress (Kanner *et al.*, 1981). These tasks may also contribute to nurses' frustration, and have consequences for mood and thereby interactions (if, say, the number of phones is restricted). Shift work may mean that once good relationships are formed, they cannot be pursued and pairings may not be possible. Patients therefore may experience several beginnings to relationships over two or three days and nurses may not

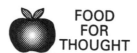

FOOD
FOR
THOUGHT

What organizational features of nursing make it easier to use effective interpersonal skills?

How does the bureaucracy of the health service affect nurses' interpersonal skills?

In what ways are nurses' interpersonal skills affected by the purchaser/provider split in the health service?

How has the introduction of the Patients' Charter influenced the interpersonal skills of nurses?

How might changes be made to the organization of nursing so that nurses could better use their interpersonal skills?

see any relationships through over the same period. Thus both are relating in unpredictable circumstances and may well feel frustrated as a result.

Many of the organizational aspects of the nursing context contribute to what we can call the **organizational culture**. Morgan (1986) suggests that 'culture' encompasses ideology, values, rituals and knowledge. Most organizations contain many different and competing value systems that create what he refers to as 'a mosaic of organizational realities, rather than a uniform corporate culture' (p. 127). Despite this, Morgan suggests that it is useful to look at the dominant culture and subcultures, as well as countercultures, in order to understand the experiences of different groups of workers. The organizational culture affects the wellbeing of the people working within it, and this in turn affects their interpersonal behaviour. Several things influence the quality of the organizational culture; for example, the amount of autonomy people are given, coupled with the degree of consideration, warmth and support they receive from their superiors will affect morale. If nurses are allowed no autonomy, or are given too much too soon, they may develop a lack of self-confidence or anxiety at the responsibility they are expected to bear. If their work is highly structured and supervised too stringently, again they may develop a lack of confidence that results in a reluctance to take decisions in conversations with patients.

There are several interesting things about the effect of organizational culture on people at work. The culture is a perceived one and not everyone will react in the same way to the same organizational context. Furthermore, people at different stages of their careers may respond differently to particular organizational practices. So, it may well be that student nurses gain confidence from highly structured and supervised work settings but more senior nurses do not. Thus the organizational culture will have different effects on different people's skills.

Since the NHS management inquiry in 1983 the culture of the health service has been evolving rapidly (DHSS, 1983). The pace of change in structure, organization and management of the health service and of nursing within it has contributed to stress for some (Hingley and Cooper, 1986). As the service has moved towards the operation of the internal market, many nurses have been redeployed and made redundant. They may or may not have had much control over the decisions. Performance criteria linked to statistical throughput of patients have been introduced, seriously undermining the value of time-consuming therapeutic relationships. Debates are still continuing about what is and is not 'nursing' – when decisions are made about 'skill mix' in the care of patients in the hospital or in the community, interpersonal skills may not feature highly in the skills required of qualified nurses. Spurgeon and Barwell (1991) map out some of the cultural changes and their implementation during the preceding decade.

When organizational culture is in transition, staff can become demoralised, frustrated, demotivated. As one respondent in Kagan and Child's (1993) study put it. 'There is little incentive to get to know our clients and help them live better lives – all they [the managers] are interested in is whether the budget is balanced.'

We have noted above that organizational factors can not only put constraints on the opportunities for interaction, but also affect the level of morale of nurses at work. The environmental context, too, can put similar constraints on the use of interpersonal skill.

ENVIRONMENTAL CONSTRAINTS

By environmental context we are referring to the physical aspects of nursing contexts and the associated rules for acting within them.

Physical environment

The physical layout of a nursing setting will encourage certain interactions and discourage others. It has been shown time and time again that if we pass others often, we are likely to talk to them (Burton, 1985). So patients near the nursing office, near doorways of the wards, near the day room, etc. are more likely to be talked to than those more distant from the amenities or the 'routes' of activity. Highly polished floors may prevent patients who are a little unsteady on their feet from finding a nurse in order to initiate conversation. (Highly polished floors or long corridors with nowhere to rest encourage patients to stay in an inactive sick role!) Nurses who spend a lot of time in the office or kitchen (with a 'Staff only' notice on the door) also limit the opportunities for interaction.

Similarly, the physical layout of the wards, day rooms, clinics and people's own homes constrains the amount and quality of interaction. It is not surprising to find nurses standing at the foot of the bed talking to bedridden patients, if all the corridors pass the bed ends. The physical distance that is maintained makes it difficult to have intimate conversations. Day rooms that have the chairs placed round the edges of the room, or facing the television or the window, make it difficult to converse with anyone but an immediate neighbour. This arrangement is typical of many settings for elderly or psychologically disabled people. It is particularly important to understand the limiting effect of the physical layout if part of patient progress is judged by the amount or quality of their interactions (as, for example, in elderly or psychiatric settings – Kagan and Burton, 1982). People's own homes can be just as obstructive to good interpersonal relations.

The style and position of furnishings is important too, affecting the feelings of the people using them (and thereby interpersonal skills).

Consider, for example, the community nurse visiting a middle-aged woman severely disabled by multiple sclerosis. She is depressed and upset about her own deteriorating condition and the effect this is having on her marriage. She does, however, try to keep herself occupied with books and simple handicrafts. As a result, her chair is surrounded by these activities, effectively creating a barrier between herself and anyone else she is talking to. Will it be possible for the nurse to get close enough to her in order to respond warmly or therapeutically? Probably not! Her/his interpersonal skills are curtailed by the physical barrier the patient has constructed around herself.

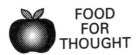
FOOD
FOR
THOUGHT

Are demanding patients the least accessible?

How do nurses compensate for the physical setting in terms of their interpersonal skills?

What effect do noise and heat have on the effective use of interpersonal skills?

What happens if a) nurses and b) patients are 'thwarted' in their control over the environment?

How does lack of privacy affect the use of interpersonal skills with patients a) in hospital and b) in their own homes? How might this be overcome?

How does a) age and b) cultural background affect patients' perception of their environments?

Control over the physical environment

In the course of our everyday lives we have areas of personal and defensible space, space that we can lay claim to, in which to put our personal possessions and, if we want to, from which to keep out other people. Newman (1972) suggested that areas of 'defensible space' are important to us all and contribute to our feelings of 'self' and of control. In hospital there are few ways that people can lay claim to any territory as their own. Furniture can rarely be arranged to create an area of defensible space around the bed; personal effects are few and patients are often discouraged from sticking cards, photos, etc. on their bedsteads. Patients – even long-stay patients – rarely have any say over the style of furniture, curtains, etc. It is generally thought that if we are unable to control our physical environment we are liable to experience distress, which in turn will serve to inhibit our usual interpersonal skills. Similarly, if rooms are too hot, too noisy or too smelly and we cannot do anything about this, we may become disgruntled, and in extreme cases experience considerable distress. It is difficult for nurses (or anyone) to be considerate if they are hot and uncomfortable, have a headache and feel nauseous.

The critical aspect of these environmental constraints is whether or not individual people have any control over them.

Consider, for example, a particular patient who moves the position of her bed, so she is better able to see out of the window. Nurses may well simply move it back again. The patient will learn that she is not able to determine where her bed will go and will feel 'thwarted'. This may end up in a dispute between patient and nurses that would otherwise not have occurred. The nurses, too, through the patient attempting to control her environment, may be 'forced' to explain why the bed must stay where it is, what the regulations or rules are, and so on. Thus the content of their interaction with the patient is being determined, indirectly, by the physical environment.

There is another way in which the physical environment affects social behaviour, and that is through what we call the **portable environment** (Kagan and Burton, 1982).

Portable environment

The portable environment refers to those movable features of a setting that tell other people something about the people involved and so go some way to determining how they behave towards these people. Let us take mental health nursing for our example. Clients are often presented to the world in ways that make it difficult for them to be accepted by others as 'ordinary people'. We are all familiar with problems of hospital clothing which frequently seems to carry the message 'This person is a mental patient', perhaps because of half-mast trousers, styles more suited to older or younger people, and so on. Nurses accompanying clients out and about may well act towards them in inappropriate ways, partly as a result of their portable environments.

Consider for example the 30-year-old woman with a learning disability who is wearing ankle socks and a baggy print dress and may be spoken to as if she were a child. Let us consider too, the signs around the hospitals (Danger: Patients Walking) or the car park of a Child Development Centre (Slow Children); uncorrected obesity; inappropriate greetings that are encouraged (people with learning disabilities who approach and want to hug complete strangers); phenothiazine gaits, and so on. What does it mean when a local Round Table advertises 'balmy boat race to raise money for handicapped children'? All these and more conspire to say damaging things about our clients and encourage certain attitudes and prejudices in nurses which constrain their use of interpersonal skill in ways that prohibit their clients from experiencing ordinary relationships.

A good example of how the content of nurse conversation can be affected by the portable environment can be seen in the following (apocryphal) story. Two nurses were taking some clients from a day centre on an outing in a minibus. The minibus was portable environment in so far as it had 'Starlight House: Hospital Day Centre for the Mentally Handicapped: Donated by Dogooders Building Society' written on both sides. This tells 'outsiders' quite a bit about the occupants both in terms of their disabilities and as objects of charity. One nurse was driving, so he could not be a client. The other might have been 'mistaken' for a client, though, so whenever he could, he spoke in such a way as to make it clear that he did not have a learning disability, just in case anyone should be watching or listening to him. The efforts he spent doing this meant that he spent very little time actually talking to clients. He was acting in this way in order to overcome the stigmatizing effects of the portable environment.

These issues do not only relate to the learning disability and mental health services, they are also relevant to other nursing settings. Health service stickers on community nurses' cars, the wearing of uniforms in the community, bars at the windows of hospitals, etc. are all examples of the portable environment that can affect attitudes and thereby interpersonal skills. Societal attitudes (nurses are part of society) and values reflect the cultural content of nursing and it is worth stopping for a moment to consider how interpersonal skills are affected by the wider social issues.

CULTURAL CONSTRAINTS

At first glance it may seem that the wider social or cultural environment can have little effect on the interpersonal skills of nurses. We will argue, though, that it does, and that the effects are widespread and can be both direct and indirect.

Ideology

We live in a society where the prevailing ideology is one of the individual control and responsibility. We are expected (and expect others) to take responsibility for, and to control, all aspects of our lives, including our health. Thus when we find that health is not within our control, the consequences are particularly traumatic and we may find ourselves in a state of 'helplessness' (Seligman, 1975), which is itself demoralizing and stressful. It is sometimes argued that physical and psychiatric illness may be a way of coping with other uncontrollable events in our lives. The emphasis on personal responsibility throughout every facet of life puts very real constraints on how nurses relate to other people.

Consider, for example, health education. Nurses are increasingly expected to fulfil a health educator role (this emphasis is in itself a direct result of policy, stemming from both governmental policies and cultural values). But what kind of health education are they encouraged to promote? It is unlikely that nurses will interpret this role as explaining/informing/teaching members of the public how governmental policies and environmental issues can have

direct consequences on everybody's health. It is instead, more
likely that they will interpret it as explaining/informing/teaching
people how they can eat, exercise, drink, look after themselves
(i.e., the Health Education's Council's propaganda scheme called
'Look After Yourself'), etc. so that their chances of enjoying good
health are increased. Given this orientation, nurses will use particular interpersonal skills in pursuit of particular goals.

Recent innovations by the Government, such as the Patients' Charter
(ACHC, 1991), *The Health of the Nation* (Department of Health, 1992),
the internal market in the health service and the changes in community
care all reflect ideological shifts that will influence nurses' interpersonal
skills. There has been a (yet to be appreciated) shift from service-led to
consumer-led health services. Consumers of health care are to participate in assessing their needs and evaluating their service. Complaints
systems have been introduced. Thus nurses are now have to encourage, receive and deal with complaints as well as trying to encourage
participation by service users. This all emphasizes interpersonal skills
in new ways (Heginbotham, 1993; Rigge and Cole, 1993). With pur-
chaser/provider splits, new requirements will be made on nurses to
explain why, for example, if they work in a community provider unit
they cannot also take part in assessments. Similarly, if they work as
care managers, they will not be providing the nursing care they have
identified is needed.

A new discourse has been introduced into health services, making its
appearance from 1980 onwards, namely that of quality and quality
assurance (Ellis and Whittingham, 1990; Nattrass, 1992; Pfeffer and
Coote, 1992). Pfeffer (1992) argues that different approaches to quality
have different implications. Scientific approaches stress statistical
monitoring and standard setting; 'excellence' approaches stress user
satisfaction and complaints; consumerist approaches stress user choice
and involvement in purchasing. Each of these approaches requires
different interpersonal emphases (on, for example, negotiation, feedback, assertion, openness to criticism, and so on). Pfeffer argues for a
new democratic approach to quality that involves meaningful participation from users and requires skills of information giving, simulation,
facilitation, support for user representatives, open channels and modes
of communication, and strategies to seek the views of those not able to
participate.

Thus, ideology both directly affects nurses' use of interpersonal skills
and indirectly affects them via governmental and professional policies.

It is worth considering what happens to the nurse when s/he meets
someone who flatly refuses either to participate in planning and
evaluating services or to follow the treatment regime recommended.

The nurse may experience conflict because another ideological force operating is that of the importance of choice and the exercise of free will. Indeed, part of the rhetoric of recent legislation makes this quite explicit. We like to think that we have choice over different aspects of our lives, but in reality we may find we do not. Nurses may experience problems in relating to people who do exercise free choice in ways that go directly against the nurse's personal stance. As nurses may now be purchasers, providers or (potential) consumers of health care, it may be useful to ask at such times 'What would I do, or how would I feel in such circumstances?'

The 'freedom of choice' issue leads into the ethical and moral contexts of nursing (Beardshaw, 1981). Nurses who try to exercise their free choice over ethical/moral issues may find themselves in direct conflict with colleagues or, indeed, with their professional bodies.

Consider, for example, the nurse who considers patient care to be put seriously at risk because of low staffing levels. He will have to use interpersonal skills of explanation, assertion, negotiation and possibly confrontation with colleagues and with professional and general managers. When he is dismissed for speaking about his concerns to the press, he will have to bring the same skills to bear in any appeal against unfair dismissal. We are seeing increasing interest in the phenomenon of 'whistle blowing' in the health service. Each instance wherein a nurse does, or is tempted to, 'blow the whistle' requires her/him to confront and challenge her/his professional ethics, and as a result employ interpersonal skills to argue her/his case or to desist from so doing.

We have seen, then, that ideology can directly curtail the interpersonal skills of nurses. It can also have indirect effects in so far as it helps determine (and is determined by) government policies and attitudes towards health care, and these in turn affect nurses' interpersonal relationships.

Government policies

The policies of different governments towards health care, and in particular the role that the National Health Service (NHS) is to play in

the delivery of that care, can affect nurses in several ways, with implications for their use of interpersonal skills. The funding of the NHS has
consequences for staffing levels and hence the opportunities to talk
with patients as well as for nurses' morale. Recent changes in the
health service, with the introduction of the internal market and the
privatizing of many parts of the service may be contradictory to nurses'
own values and political beliefs (Higgs, 1993). Nurses who find themselves participating in discussions and strategies about the transfor-
mation of their part of the service into an NHS trust, when they are
politically opposed to such trusts, may have difficulty negotiating effectively. On the other hand, those that are sympathetic to the changes
may find new opportunities to develop and use interpersonal skills
required in managing the new organizations (Stamp, 1992). The plu-
rality of purchasing arrangements currently in place, affecting people
in different localities differently, may mean that it is difficult for a
nurse to reply honestly to a patient's plea 'Can nothing be done?' This
is especially so when s/he believes that there might have been some
hope, if specialist service had not been cut or purchasing arrangements
had been different. These types of effect are different for different care
groups, as priority areas are identified.

The NHS and Community Care Act (HMSO, 1990) has transformed
the care of vulnerable and dependent people. There are incentives to
support people in their own homes as long as possible. This may mean
that resources are transferred from hospital to community and that the
pattern of nursing services being purchased will change, requiring
nurses to change how they work. Depending on local care management arrangements, community nurses may or may not take part in
the assessment of need. Certainly there will be greater emphasis in the
future on interdisciplinary assessment and provision, highlighting the
need for interpersonal collaboration and teamwork, as well as the skills
involved in helping consumers participate, and in user empowerment
(Winn, 1990).

Restructuring the NHS affects nurses' morale every time it occurs,
as they are repeatedly asked to work in the context of considerable
personal insecurity.

The privatization of health care, and support of the pharmaceutical
industry both help to create a tension in the need to make profits out of
health care. Nurses may find themselves compromised in various ways
or subject to massive advertising and propaganda campaigns which
restrict their decision-making processes, and may well then influence
what advice they give patients (although of course, we all like to
believe that we are not open to such influences!).

There are many other ways that government policies can have effects
on the interpersonal skills of nurses, but these examples should serve
to illustrate the point. Both government and prevailing ideologies

directly influence the interpersonal skills of nurses: they also influence the professional bodies concerned with nursing.

Professional nursing bodies

It is the professional bodies that prescribe the role of the nurse in the general and specific training syllabi for the various specialisms. Thus they determine the professional attitude towards the importance of interpersonal skills, and hence the amount of time spent in training and the serious consideration that should be paid to these aspects of nursing. Recently, Project 2000 has been introduced, which has changed the nature and structure of initial nurse training and of the colleges of health that deliver the courses. This has led to a number of pressures that militate against being able to teach interpersonal skills in a sensitive and individually focused way.

Many initial nurse training courses are now teaching far larger groups of students than they did before, which presents a major challenge to interpersonal skills teaching. It is impossible with large groups to give individual attention to students' progress. This can mean that the teaching becomes more 'academic' rather than experiential and that anything that might be personally sensitive is avoided. However, it may also mean that tutors have to learn to let go of student learning and to build on techniques that encourage students in autonomous learning and in the tracking of their own progress.

As more students enter nurse training from schools wherein they have compiled records of achievement, including core transferable academic skills such as communication and problem solving, they will themselves be in a position to pressurize nurse educators to allow them to build on their self-monitoring capabilities. Similarly, students are about to offer National Vocational Qualifications (NVQs) and General National Vocational Qualifications (GNVQs) as entry qualifications to nurse training, and these emphasize capability in communication, problem solving and group or team work. These different experiences and capabilities of students entering nurse training will mean that teachers will have to adopt flexible teaching strategies that allow different students to develop at their own pace.

Currently, the English National Board and the United Kingdom Central Council for Nursing and Midwifery and Health Visiting all concede the importance of interpersonal skills as a vital nursing skill. Nevertheless, the relative importance varies with the type of nursing. Different syllabi, however, give different weight to interpersonal skills in comparison with other nursing skills. It is up to training bodies to prioritize interpersonal skills: if they do not it is unlikely that practising nurses will do so.

In this section we have discussed some of the features of the social or cultural context of nursing which can impose direct or indirect constraints on nurses' use of interpersonal skills.

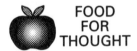

FOOD FOR THOUGHT

How does the internal market in the health service influence nursing practice?

What interpersonal skills are required of nurses as (a) commissioners, (b) providers of health care?

How many restructures of the health service have there been since 1980? What direct or indirect effect have these had on nursing?

What taboos are there in this society connected to health and illness? How have they come about?

What impact do nurses' own values and political beliefs have on their ability to make effective use of interpersonal skills?

What roles do nurses have in bringing about political and social change?

What interpersonal skills are involved in a) advocacy, b) 'whistle blowing', c) multidisciplinary teamwork and d) care management?

How adequate are interpersonal skills components of professional training courses in preparing nurses to work in contemporary health services?

It is only with such awareness that nurses can realistically understand and appraise their own interpersonal skills, a notion that further supports the need for all nurses to work towards increasing their own self-awareness.

SUMMARY

This chapter has focused on the context of interpersonal skills used by nurses. Specifically, the following points were raised.

- The effective use of interpersonal skills depends on the personal, social, environmental and cultural contexts in which they are deployed.
- Nurses must be able to recognize the constraints on their effective

use of interpersonal skills before they can devise strategies to overcome them.

- One-to-one therapeutic relationships with patients arouse emotions in nurses.
- Nurses' inability to express their emotions within their professional role may lead to feelings of powerlessness and low morale.
- Emotion, stress and low morale may all distort the use of interpersonal skills.
- Intimate relationships between nurses and patients develop in peculiar ways, and are unlike other relationships.
- Personal support and supervision systems are necessary as a means of helping nurses to become more self-aware, to deal constructively with their personal feelings and the pressures of work and to continue to deliver good patient care.
- The interaction context both enables and hinders effective use of interpersonal skills.
- Nurses occupy a role that is at the boundary between a number of other roles and this causes pressure.
- Nurses do not like all patients equally and this will have a deleterious effect on their interpersonal skills unless they are aware of their preferences.
- Regulations applied to nursing practice can have unintended deleterious effects on the use of interpersonal skills.
- Organizational and bureaucratic procedures constrain the opportunities for and channels of effective interpersonal relationships.
- Organizational culture affects the wellbeing of those working within it.
- Nurses at different stages of their careers respond to the same organizational pressures differently.
- The introduction of the internal market in the health service has resulted in massive organizational change and turmoil for individual nurses.
- Organizational transition can demoralize staff.
- Physical environments can inhibit the use of particular interpersonal skills.
- Lack of control over the physical environment can lead to feelings of powerlessness and stress.
- Portable environments help determine and maintain attitudes and prejudices and distort the use of interpersonal skills.
- Cultural ideologies that stress individual control and responsibility can influence interpersonal skills and nurses' responses to changing work situations, in which they find themselves out of control of events.
- Consumer-focused health services will place demands on nurses to use their interpersonal skills differently.

- Many cultural changes at local and government levels result in nurses feeling despondent because they feel de-skilled.
- The recent emphasis on 'quality' and consumer participation in health care will require a change in emphasis in nurses' interpersonal behaviour towards more openness to complaints and feedback, greater collaboration and the use of facilitation skills.
- Ideology surrounds the ethical and moral dilemmas faced by nurses and these can have indirect consequences for their use of interpersonal skills.
- Government policies and attitudes towards nurses can indirectly affect their morale and use of interpersonal skills.
- Professional bodies are influenced by government and prevailing ideology. They in turn prescribe the status given to interpersonal skills in the training and practice of nurses.
- Changes in nurse training stand in danger of devaluing experiential approaches to the learning and development of interpersonal skills in favour of academic knowledge about interpersonal skills.

SELF-DEVELOPMENT EXERCISES

1. Think of a patient you like a lot and one that you do not like much. What is the difference between them? How much in common do you have with either of them? How do you and your colleagues compensate for disliking a patient?
2. Write a letter to an imaginary friend who know nothing about nursing. Try to describe the pleasant and unpleasant aspects of the job. Include some mention of how you cope with the pressures and where you get personal support from. Be as specific as you can about the kinds of support you get and how this helps you manage.
3. Interview a student nurse soon after s/he has spent the first few days in contact with patients as a nurse. Find out how s/he felt about actually doing nursing and how the behaviour of others around her/him (colleagues, other medical and paramedical personnel, patients, relatives, and so on) either helped her/him fulfil her/his role or not.
4. Imagine you are writing a practitioners' manual for those doing your job. What headings would you include under the section 'Regulations'? What impact do these regulations have on your use of interpersonal skills?
5. Draw a map of the place where you work. Mark on the map those areas that would be difficult to negotiate in a wheelchair; those areas with restricted access; those areas where certain behaviours are proscribed (for example, smoking, eating). Look now at your official site map. Are any of these restrictions marked on it?

6. Identify features of the portable environment you carry about with you. How might anyone else know you are a nurse? When you are out and about, try to detect features of some portable environments of health service users (this will be especially easy for people with physical impairments, mental health problems, learning disabilities and elderly people). How might these portable environments convey more positive messages to the 'outside' world?

7. Read a national newspaper every day for a month. Take cuttings of all articles concerned with health or health care. What assumptions are made in them about people who use health services, those who work in them, those who manage them and those who create the policies that guide them? What ideologies and values underpin the articles you have collected? Are they beneficial to those who use and work in the health service or not?

8. Devise an advertisement 'selling' your particular nursing service to a potential purchaser. Try to focus on the positive achievements of the service in the context of recent health service change. When you have done this, consider how realistic it is, and how the situation you have described might be reached.

References

ACHC (1991) *From Citizens' Charter to Patients' Charter*, Association of CHCs of England and Wales, London.

Adair, J. (1983) *Effective Leadership*, Pan, London.

Adair, J. (1984a) *Action-Centred Leadership*, Gower, Aylesbury.

Adair, J. (1984b) *The Skills of Leadership*, Gower, Aylesbury.

Adams, J., Hayes, J. and Hopson, B. (eds) (1976) *Transition: Understanding and Managing Personal Change*, Martin Robertson, London.

Adams, M.L. (1989) There's no place like home: on the place of identity in feminist politics *Feminist Review*, **31**, 22–33.

Ajzen, I. and Madden, T.J. (1986) Prediction of goal directed behavior: attitudes, intentions and perceived behavioral control *Journal of Experimental Social Psychology*, **22**, 453–474.

Antaki, C. (ed.) (1981) *The Psychology of Ordinary Explanations of Social Behaviour*, Academic Press, London.

Antaki, C. (ed.) (1988) *Analysing Everyday Explanation: A Casebook of Methods*, Sage Publications, London.

Argyle, M. (1983) *The Psychology of Interpersonal Behaviour*, 4th edn, Penguin, Harmondsworth.

Argyle, M. (1986) Social skills and the analysis of situations and conversations, in *Handbook of Social Skills Training 2: Clinical Applications and New Directions*, (eds C.R. Hollin and P. Trower), Pergamon Press, Oxford.

Argyle, M., Furnham, A. and Graham, J. (1981) *Social Situations*, Cambridge University Press, Cambridge.

Argyle, M. and Henderson, M. (1985) *The Anatomy of Relationships*, Penguin, Harmondsworth.

Asch, S. (1946) Forming impressions of personality. *Journal of Abnormal and Social Psychology*, **41**, 258–290.

Bailey, R. and Clarke, M. (1989) *Stress and Coping in Nursing*, Chapman & Hall, London.

Bales, R.F. (1950) A set of categories for the analysis of small group interaction *American Sociological Review*, **15**, 257–263.

Bandura, A. (1977) *Social Learning Theory*, Prentice Hall, Englewood Cliffs, NJ.

Bandura, A. (1978) The self system in reciprocal determinism. *American Psychologist*, **33**, 344–358.

Bandura, A. (1986) *Social Foundations of Thought and Action*, Prentice Hall, Englewood Cliffs, NJ.

Bannister, D. and Fransella, F. (1989) *Inquiring Man*, 3rd edn, Penguin, Harmondsworth.

Barber, P. (1989) Developing the 'person' of the professional carer, in *Nursing Practice and Health Care*, (eds S. Hinchliff, S. Norman and J. Schober), Edward Arnold, London.

Bartlett, F. (1932) *Remembering*, Cambridge University Press, Cambridge.

Beardshaw, V. (1981) *Conscientious Objectors at Work: Mental Hospital Nurses – A Case Study*, Social Audit, London.

Becker, M.H. and Maiman, L.A. (1980) Strategies for enhancing patient compliance. *Journal of Community Health*, **6**, 113–135.

Becker, M.H., Maiman, L.A., Kirscht, J.P. *et al.* (1979) Patient perceptions and compliance: recent studies of the health belief model, in *Compliance in Health Care*, (eds R.B. Haynes, D.W. Taylor and D.L. Sackett), Johns Hopkins University Press, Baltimore, MD.

Belbin, R.M. (1981) *Management Teams: Why They Succeed or Fail*, Butterworth-Heinemann, Oxford.

Benne, K.D. and Sheats, P. (1948) Functional roles of group members. *Journal of Social Issues*, **4**, 41–49.

Berkowitz, L. (1969) The frustration–aggression hypothesis revisited, in *Roots of Aggression*, (ed. L. Berkowitz), Atherton: New York.

Berkowitz, L. (1983) The experience of anger as a parallel process in the display of impulsive, 'angry' aggression, in *Aggression: Theoretical and Empirical Reviews*, vol. 1, (eds R.G. Green and E.I. Donnerstein), Academic Press, New York.

Berne, E. (1964) *Games People Play*, Grove Press, New York.

Berne, E. (1974) *What Do You Say After You Say 'Hello'?*, Grove Press, New York.

Billig, M., Condor, S., Edwards, D. *et al.* (1988) *Ideological Dilemmas: A Social Psychology of Everyday Thinking*, Sage Publications, London.

Billings, A.G. and Moos, R.H. (1981) The role of coping responses and social resources in attenuating the stress of life events. *Journal of Behavioral Medicine*, **4**, 139–157.

Bochner, S. (ed.) (1981) *Cultures in Contact*, Pergamon Press, Oxford.

Bond, M. (1986) *Stress and Self-Awareness: A Guide for Nurses*, Heinemann, London.

Booth, T.A. (1978) From normal baby to handicapped child. *Sociology*, **12**, 203–221.

Bottom, W.D. (1987) Physician assistants: current status of the profession. *Journal of Family Practice*, **24**, 7639–7644.

Bowles, L. (1991) Journey through fear. *Nursing Times*, **87**(8), 44–45.

Boyd, J. (1978) *Counsellor Supervision: Approaches, Preparation and Practices*, Accelerated Development, Muncie, IN.

Brandon, D. and Brandon, A. (1987) *Consumers as Colleagues*, MIND, London.

Breakwell, G. (1986) *Coping with Threatened Identities*, Methuen, London.

Brewer, M.B. and Kramer, R.M. (1985) The psychology of intergroup attitudes and behaviour. *Annual Review of Psychology*, **36**, 219–243.

Brown, G. and Harris, T. (eds) (1978) *The Social Origins of Depression*, Tavistock, London.

Brown, G. and Harris, T. (eds) (1989) *Life Events and Illness*, Guilford Press, New York.

Brown, R. (1988) *Group Processes: Dynamics Within and Between Groups*, Blackwell, Oxford.

Bruner, J.S. and Tagiuri, R. (1954) The perception of people, in *Handbook of Social Psychology*, vol. 2, (ed. G. Lindzey), Addison Wesley, Cambridge, MA.

Burchfield, S.R. (ed.) (1985) *Stress: Psychological and Physiological Interactions*, Hemisphere, Washington, DC.

Burnard, P. (1989) *Counselling Skills for Health Professionals*, Chapman & Hall, London.

Burton, M. (1980) Evaluation and change in a psychogeriatric ward through direct observation and feedback. *British Journal of Psychiatry*, **137**, 566–571.

Burton, M. (1985) The environment, good interactions and interpersonal skills in nursing, in *Interpersonal Skills in Nursing: Research and Applications*, (ed. C. Kagan), Croom Helm, London.

Burton, M. (1991) *Caught in the Competence Trap*, Regional Advisory Group for Learning Disability Services, North Western Regional Health Authority, Manchester.

Burton, M. (1992) *Roads to Quality*, Regional Advisory Group for Learning Disability Services, North Western Regional Health Authority, Manchester.

Buss, A.H. (1980) *Self Consciousness and Social Anxiety*, W. & H. Freeman, New York.

Butterworth, C.A. and Faugier, J. (eds) (1992) *Clinical Supervision and Mentorship in Nursing*, Chapman & Hall, London.

Caine, N. (1993) Heart to heart: the role of transplant clinician assistants. *Health Services Journal*, **16 Sept.**, 22–24.

Campling, J. (1981) *Images of Ourselves: Women with Disabilities Talking*, Routledge & Kegan Paul, London.

Carkhuff, R. (1983) *The Art of Helping*, Holt, Rinehart & Winston, New York.

Carter, W.B. (1990) Health behavior as a rational process: theory of reasoned action and multi-attribute utility theory, in *Health Behavior and Health Education: Theory, Research and Practice*, (eds K. Glanz, F.M. Lewis and B.K. Rimer), Jossey Bass, San Francisco, CA.

Chadwick-Jones, J.K. (1976) *Social Exchange Theory*, Academic Press, London.

Challela, M.S. (1981) Helping parents cope with a profoundly mentally retarded child, in *Coping With Crisis and Handicap*, (ed. A. Mulinsky), Plenum Press, New York.

Cherniss, C. and Egnatios, E. (1978) Clinical supervision in community mental health. *Social Work* (London), **23/2**, 219–223.

Clark, H. and Clark, E. (1977) *Psychology and Language: An Introduction to Psycholinguistics*, Harcourt Brace Jovanovich, New York.

Claus, K.E. and Bailey, J.T. (eds) (1980) *Living with Stress and Promoting Well Being: A Handbook for Nurses*, C.V. Mosby, St Louis, MO.

Cohen, F. (1988) *Life Events and Functioning*, Sage Publications, New York.

Cohen, S. and McKay, G. (1984) Social support, stress and the buffering hypothesis: a theoretical analysis, in *Handbook of Psychology and Health*, (eds A. Baum, S.E. Taylor and J.E. Singer), Lawrence Erlbaum Associates, Hillsdale, NJ.

Cooley, C.H. (1902) *Human Nature and the Social Order*, Charles Scribner, New York.

Cooper, J. and Fazio, R.H. (1984) A new look at dissonance theory, in *Advances in Experimental Social Psychology 17*, (ed. L. Berkowitz), Academic Press, New York.

Copp, G. (1988) The reality behind stress. *Nursing Times*, **84**(45), 50–53.

Cormack, D. (1985) The myth and reality of interpersonal skills in nursing, in *Interpersonal Skills in Nursing: Research and applications*, (ed. C. Kagan), Croom Helm, London.

Cox, T. (1978) *Stress*, Macmillan, London.

Croft, S. and Beresford, P. (1990) *From Paternalism to Participation: Involving people in local services*, Open Services Project/Joseph Rowntree Foundation, York.

Crossland, J. (1992) Training nurses to deal with aggressive encounters with the public. University of Oxford. Unpublished DPhil thesis.

Crotty, M. (1987) 'Burnout' and its implications for the continuing education of nurses. *Nurse Education Today*, **7**, 278–284.

Cuff, T., Sharrock, W. and Francis, D. (1992) *Perspectives in Sociology*, 3rd edn, Routledge, London.

Cullen, C., Burton, M., Watts, S. and Thomas, M. (1983) A preliminary report on the nature of interactions in a mental handicap institution. *Behaviour, Research and Therapy*, **21**, 579–583.

Dainow, S. and Bailey, C. (1988) *Developing Skills with People: Training for Person to Person Client Contact*, John Wiley, Chichester.

Dale, N., Sklavounos, D., Specker, N. and Wiseman, G. (1991) *Shared Concern: Breaking the News to Parents that Their Child Has a Disability*, 3rd edn, SOPHIE, Kings Fund Centre, London.

Davis, B. (1985) The clinical effect of interpersonal skills: the implementation of pre-operative information giving, in *Interpersonal Skills in Nursing: Research and Applications*, (ed. C. Kagan), Croom Helm, London.

Dewe, P. (1991) Primary appraisal, secondary appraisal and coping: their role in stressful work encounters *Journal of Occupational Psychology*, **64**, 331–351.

Department of Health (1992) *The Health of the Nation*, HMSO, London.

DHSS (Department of Health and Social Security) (1983) *National Health Service Management Enquiry (the Griffiths Report)*, HMSO, London.

Dickson, A. (1982) *A Woman in Your Own Right: Assertiveness and You*, Quartet Books, London.

Dickson, D. (1986) Reflecting, in *A Handbook of Communication Skills*, (ed. O. Hargie), Croom Helm, London.

Dickson, D., Saunders, C. and Stringer, M. (1993) *Rewarding People: The Skill of Responding Positively*, Routledge, London.

Diener, E. (1980) Deindividuation: the absence of self-awareness and self-regulation in group members, in *The Psychology of Group Influence*, (ed. P. Paulus), Lawrence Erlbaum Associates, Hillsdale, NJ.

Dillon, J.T. (1990) *The Practice of Questioning*, Routledge, London.

DiMatteo, M.R. and DiNicola, D.D. (1982) *Achieving Patient Compliance*, Pergamon Press, New York.

DiNicola, D.D. and DiMatteo, M.R. (1982) Communication, interpersonal influence and resistance to medical treatment, in *Basic Processes in Helping Relationships*, (ed. T.A. Willis), Academic Press, New York.

DiNicola, D.D. and DiMatteo, M.R. (1984) Practitioners, patients and compliance with medical regimes: a social psychological perspective, in *Handbook of Psychology and Health*, (eds A. Baum, S.E. Taylor and J.E. Singer) Lawrence Erlbaum Associates, Hillsdale, NJ.

Dolan, C. (1987) The relationship between burnout and job satisfaction in nursing. *Journal of Advanced Nursing*, **12**, 3–12.

Drucker, P. (1980) *Managing in Turbulent Times*, Harper & Row, New York.

Durkin, K. (1988) The social nature of social development, in *Introduction to Social Psychology*, (eds M. Hewstone, W. Stroebe, J.-P. Codol and G.M. Stephenson), Blackwell, Oxford.

Duval, S. and Wicklund, R.A. (1972) *A Theory of Objective Self-Awareness*, Academic Press, New York.

D'Zurilla, T.J. and Nezu, A. (1982) Social problem solving in adults, in *Advances in Cognitive Behavioral Research and Therapy*, (ed. P.C. Kendall), Academic Press, New York.

Egan, G. (1986) *The Skilled Helper*, 3rd edn, Brookes/Cole, Monterey, CA.

Ehrenfeld, M. and Cheifetz, F.R. (1990) Cardiac nurses: coping with stress. *Journal of Advanced Nursing*, **15**, 1002–1008.

Eiser, R. (1980) *Cognitive Social Psychology* McGraw Hill, London.

Eiser, R. (1986) *Social Psychology: Attitudes, Cognition and Social Behaviour*, Cambridge University Press, Cambridge.

Ekman, P. and Friesen, W.V. (1969) Non-verbal leakage and clues to deception. *Psychiatry*, **32**, 88–1096.

Ekman, P., Friesen, W.V. and Ancoli, S. (1980) Facial signs of emotional experience. *Journal of Personality and Social Psychology*, **39**, 1125–1134.

Elliott, G.R. and Eisdorfer, C. (eds) (1982) *Stress and Human Health*, Springer, New York.

Ellis, R. and Whittingham, D. (1993) *Quality Assurance in Health Care: A Handbook*, Edward Arnold, London.

Epting, T.R. (1984) *Personal Construct Counselling and Psychotherapy*, John Wiley, Chichester.

Erickson, E.H. (1950) *Childhood, Self and Society*, Norton, New York.

Errington, G. (1989) Stress among disaster nurses and relief workers. *International Nursing Review*, **36**(3), 90–91.

Estabrooks, C.A. (1987) Touch in nursing practice: a historical perspective. *Journal of Nursing History*, **2**(2), 33–49.

Estabrooks, C.A. and Morse, J.M. (1992) Towards a theory of touch: the touching process and acquiring a touching style. *Journal of Advanced Nursing*, **17**, 448–456.

Fanon, F. (1986) *Black Skins, White Masks*, Pluto Press, London.

Faugier, J. (1991) Don't do as I do . . . *Nursing Times*, **87**(15), 32.

Faulkner, A. (1985) The organisational context of interpersonal skills in nursing, in *Interpersonal Skills in Nursing: Research and Applications*, (ed. C. Kagan), Croom Helm, London.

Fazio, R.H. and Zanna, M.P. (1981) Direct experience and attitude-behavior consistency, in *Advances in Experimental Social Psychology 14*, (ed. L. Berkowitz), Academic Press, New York, pp. 161–202.

Felner, R.D., Farber, S.S. and Primavera, J. (1985) Transitions and stressful life events: a model for primary prevention, in *Preventive Psychology*, (eds R.D. Felner, L.A. Jason, J.N. Moritsugu and S.S. Farber), Pergamon Press, New York.

Festinger, L. (1954) A theory of social comparison processes. *Human Relations*, **7**, 117–140.

Festinger, L. (1957) *A Theory of Cognitive Dissonance*, Stanford University Press, Stanford, CA.

Fiedler, F.E. (1950) The concept of an ideal therapeutic relationship. *Journal of Consulting Psychology*, **14**, 239–245.

Fiedler, F.E. (1976) *Improving Leadership Effectiveness: The Leader Match Context*, John Wiley, New York.

Field, D. (1984) 'We didn't want him to die on his own' – nurses' accounts of nursing dying patients. *Journal of Advanced Nursing*, **9**, 59–70.

Firth, H., McIntee, J., McKeown, P. and Britton, P. (1985) Maslach burnout inventory: factor structure and norms for British nursing staff. *Psychological Reports*, **57**(1), 147–152.

Firth, H., McIntee, J., McKeown, P. and Britton, P. (1986) Interpersonal support amongst nurses at work. *Journal of Advanced Nursing*, **11**(3), 273–282.

Fishbein, M. and Ajzen, I. (1975) *Belief, Attitude, Intention and Behavior: An Introduction to Theory and Research*, Addison-Wesley, Reading, MA.

Fisher, R. and Ury, W. (1981) *Getting to Yes: Negotiating Agreement Without Giving In*, Houghton Mifflin, Boston, MA.

Fiske, S.T. and Taylor, S.E. (1984) *Social Cognition*, Random House, New York.

Fiske, S.T. and Taylor, S.E. (1991) *Social Cognition*, 2nd edn, Random House, New York.

Forgas, J. (1985a) *Interpersonal Behaviour*, Pergamon Press, Oxford.

Forgas, J. (ed.) (1985b) *Language and Social Situations*, Springer, New York.

Forgas, J.P., O'Connor, K. and Morris, S. (1983) Smile and punishment: the effects of facial expression on responsibility attribution by groups and individuals. *Personality and Social Psychology Bulletin*, **9**, 587–596.

Forsyth, D. (1983) *An Introduction to Group Dynamics*, Brooks/Cole, Monterey, CA.

Freeman, J. (1970) The tyranny of structurelessness, in *Untying the Knot: Feminism, Anarchism and Organization* Dark Star Press and Rebel Press, London.

French, J.R.P. (1964) A formal theory of social power. *Psychological Review*, **63**, 181–194.

French, J.R.P. and Raven, B.H. (1959) The bases of social power, in *Studies in Social Power*, (ed. D. Cartwright), University of Michigan Press, Ann Arbor, MI.

French, P. (1983) *Social Skills for Nursing Practice*, Croom Helm, London.

Friedman, S. and Rosenman, R.H. (1974) *Type A Behavior and Your Heart*, Knopf, New York.

Gahagan, J. (1984) *Social Interaction and its Management*, Methuen, London.

Gaze, H. (1988) Stressed to the limit. *Nursing Times*, **84**(36), 16–17.

George, V. and Wilding, P. (1985) *Ideology and Social Welfare*, Routledge & Kegan Paul, London.

Gergen, K.J. (1985) The social constructionist movement in modern psychology. *American Psychologist*, **40**, 266–275.

Gergen, K.J., Morse, S.J. and Gergen, M.M. (1980) Behavior exchange in cross cultural perspective, in *Handbook of Cross-Cultural Psychology, vol. 5: Social Psychology*, (eds H.C. Triandis and W.W. Lambert), Allyn & Bacon, Boston, MA.

Gibson, T. (1979) *People Power: Community and Work Groups in Action*, Pelican, Harmondsworth.

Gildea, E.F. (1949) Special features of personality which are common to certain psychosomatic disorders. *Psychosomatic Medicine*, **11**, 273–281.

Glaser, B.G. and Strauss, A.L. (1965) *Awareness of Dying*, Weidenfeld & Nicholson, London.

Glasman, D. (1993) It takes one to know one: ambulance staff are becoming stress-spotters. *Health Services Journal*, **4 Nov.**, 16.

Glass, D.C. and Singer, J.E. (1972) *Urban Stress*, Academic Press, New York.

Goffman, E. (1959) *Presentation of Self in Everyday Life*, Anchor Books, New York.

Goffman, E. (1963) *Stigma: Notes on the Management of Spoiled Identity*, Prentice Hall, Englewood Cliffs, NJ.

Goffman, E. (1967) *Interaction Ritual: Essays on Face-to-Face Behaviour*, Allen Lane/Penguin Press, London.

Goffman, E. (1971) *Relations in Public: Micro-Studies of the Public Order*, Basic Books, New York.

Goldberg, E.L. and Comstock, G.W. (1980) Epidemiology of life events: frequency in general populations. *American Journal of Epidemiology*, **111**(6), 736–752.

Goldstein, A.P. and Keller, H.R. (1986) *Aggressive Behaviour: Assessment and Intervention*, Pergamon Press, New York.

Goody, E. (ed.) (1985) *Questions in Politeness: Strategies in Social Interaction,* Cambridge University Press, Cambridge.

Gould, B. (1990) Empathy: A review of the literature with suggestion for an alternative research strategy. *Journal of Advanced Nursing,* **15**, 1167–1174.

Gow, K. (1982) *How Nurses' Emotions Affect Patient Care,* Springer, New York.

Gowins-Rubin, J. (1990) Critical incident stress de-briefing: helping the helpers. *Journal of Emergency Nursing,* **16**(4), 255–258.

Graesser, A. and Black, J. (eds) (1985) *The Psychology of Questions,* Lawrence Erlbaum Associates, Hillsdale, NJ.

Hacking, M. (1981) Communication, dying and bereavement. *Nursing* (Oxford), **1**, 1168–1170.

Hallett, C. (1987) *Critical Issues in Participation,* Association of Community Workers, London.

Halliday, M.A.K. (1973) *Explorations in the Functions of Language,* Edward Arnold, London.

Hargie, O., Saunders, C. and Dickson, D. (1981) *Social Skills in Interpersonal Communication,* Croom Helm, London.

Harré, R. (1979) *Social Being,* Blackwell, Oxford.

Harré, R. (1984) *Personal Being: A theory for individual psychology,* Blackwell, Oxford.

Harré, R. (ed.) (1986) *The Social Construction of Emotions,* Blackwell, Oxford.

Harré, R. (1993) *Social Being,* 2nd edn, Blackwell, Oxford.

Harré, R. and Secord, P.F. (1972) *The Explanation of Social Behaviour,* Blackwell, Oxford.

Harvey, P. (1989) Stress and health, in *Health Psychology: Process and Applications,* (ed. A. Broome), Chapman & Hall, London.

Hawkins, L. (1987) An ergonomic approach to stress. *International Journal of Nursing Studies,* **24**(4), 307–318.

Hawkins, P. and Shohet, R. (1989) *Supervision in the Helping Professions,* Open University Press, Milton Keynes.

Hawthorne, L. (1975) Games supervisors play. *Social Work* (London), **20 May**, 179–183.

Hayward, J. (1975) *Information: a Prescription Against Pain,* Royal College of Nursing, London.

Heginbotham, C. (ed.) (1993) *Listening to Local Voices,* NAHAT, London.

Heron, J (1975) *Six Category Intervention Analysis,* University of Surrey, Human Potential Research Project, Guildford.

Hersey, P. and Blanchard, K. (1988) *Management of Organizational Behavior,* 5th edn, Prentice Hall, Englewood Cliffs, NJ.

Herzlich, C. (1974) *Health and Illness: A Social Psychological Analysis,* Academic Press, London.

Hewstone, M. and Antaki, C. (1988) Attribution theory and social explanations, in *Introduction to Social Psychology,* (eds M. Hewstone, W. Stroebe, J.-P. Codol and G.M. Stephenson), Blackwell, Oxford.

Higgs, P. (1993) *The NHS and Ideological Conflict,* Avebury, Aldershot.

Hingley, P. and Cooper, C.L. (1986) *Stress and the Nurse Manager,* John Wiley, Chichester.

Hiscox, C. (1991) Stress and its management. *Nursing Standard,* **5**(21), 36–40.

HMSO (1990) *NHS and Community Care Act,* HMSO, London.

Hogg, M. and Abrams, D. (1988) *Social Identifications: A Social Psychology of Intergroup Relations and Group Processes,* Routledge, London.

Hollin, C.R. and Trower, P. (1986a) Social skills training: critique and future directions, in *Handbook of Social Skills Training 2: Clinical Applications and New Directions*, (eds C.R. Hollin and P. Trower), Pergamon Press, Oxford.

Hollin, C.R. and Trower, P. (1986b) (eds) *Handbook of Social Skills Training 1: Applications Across the Lifespan*, Pergamon Press, Oxford.

Holmes, T.H. and Rahe, R.H. (1967) The social readjustment rating scale. *Journal of Psychosomatic Research*, **11**, 213–218.

Howden, C. and Levison, A. (1987) Coping with stress – sharing and learning. *Senior Nurse*, 7(2), 6–8.

Hughes, J. (1980) Manipulation: a negative element in care. *Journal of Advanced Nursing*, **5**, 21–29.

Hunt, M. (1991) Being friendly and informal: reflected in nurses', teminally ill patients', and relatives' conversations at home. *Journal of Advanced Nursing*, **16**, 929–938.

Hunt, P. (1986) 'Supervision'. *Marriage Guidance*, **Spring**, 15–22.

Inui, I.S. and Carter, W.B. (1985) Problems and prospects for health services research on provider–patient communication. *Medical Care*, **23**, 521–538.

Jacobson, S.F. and McGrath, H.M. (1983) *Nurses Under Stress*, John Wiley, Chichester.

Johnson, D.W. (1986) *Reaching Out: Interpersonal Effectiveness and Self Actualization*, 3rd edn, Prentice Hall, Englewood Cliffs, NJ.

Jones, S.E. and Yarbrough, A.E. (1985) A naturalistic study of the meanings of touch. *Communication Monographs*, **52**, 19–56.

Jongeward, D. (1976) *Everybody Wins: Transactional Analysis Applied to Organizations*, Addison Wesley, Reading, MA.

Jongeward, D. and James, M. (1981) *Winning Ways in Health Care: Transactional Analysis for Effective Communication*, Addison Wesley, Reading, MA.

Jourard, S. (1964) *The Transparent Self*, Van Nostrand, Princeton, NJ.

Jourard, S. (1971) *Self-Disclosure: An Experimental Study of the Transparent Self*, John Wiley, New York.

Kadushin, A. (1968) Games people play in supervision. *Social Work* (USA), **13**.

Kadushin, A. (1976) *Supervision in Social Work*, Columbia University Press, New York.

Kagan, C. (1981) Cognitive aspects of social skills training. University of Oxford. Unpublished DPhil thesis.

Kagan, C. (1982) Barriers to the effective use of interpersonal skills in the community. Paper presented to conference on Interpersonal Skills in Nursing, Manchester Polytechnic, Manchester.

Kagan, C. (1984) Social problem solving and social skills training. *British Journal of Clinical Psychology*, **23**, 161–173.

Kagan, C. (1985) Issues arising from teaching interpersonal skills in post-basic nurse training, in *Interpersonal Skills in Nursing: Research and Applications*, (ed. C. Kagan), Croom Helm, London.

Kagan, C. (1990) *What Do We Know About Care Management?*, North Western Training and Development Team, Whalley, Lancashire.

Kagan, C. (1991) The effect of others on our behaviour, in *A Textbook of Psychology*, (eds J. Radford and E. Govier), 2nd edn, Routledge, London.

Kagan, C. (1992) *Hostel Closures: Quality Contracts for Service Change*, North Western Training and Development Team, Whalley, Lancashire.

Kagan, C. (1993) *Quality of Services: The Role of Supervision in Achieving Positive Outcomes for People Using Services*, North Western Training and Development Team, Whalley, Lancashire.

Kagan, C. and Burton, M. (1982) Scenes of improvement. *Nursing Mirror*, **155**, 44–45.

Kagan, C. and Child, M. (1993) *Working Under Pressure: Good Practice for the*

Management of Stress, North Western Training and Development Team, Whalley, Lancashire.

Kagan, C., Evans, J. and Kay, B. (1986) *A Manual of Interpersonal Skills for Nurses: An Experiential Approach*, Harper & Row, London.

Kagan, N. (1979) Interpersonal skills and health care, in *Health Psychology*, (eds G.C. Stone, F. Cohen and N.E. Adler), Jossey Bass, New York.

Kanner, A.D., Coyne, J.C., Schaefer, C. and Lazarus, R.S. (1981) Comparison of two modes of stress measurement: daily hassles and uplifts versus major life events. *Journal of Behavioral Medicine*, **4**, 1–39.

Kaplan, R.M., Sallis, J.F. and Patterson, T.L. (1993) *Health and Human Behavior*, McGraw Hill, New York.

Kasl, S. (1983) Pursuing the link between stressful life events and disease: a time for appraisal, in *Stress Research: Issues for the Eighties*, (ed. C. Cooper), John Wiley, Chichester.

Kasl, S.V. and Cooper, C.L. (eds) (1987) *Stress and Health: Issues in Research Methodology*, John Wiley, Chichester.

Kennedy, E. (1977) *On Becoming a Counsellor*, Gill & Macmillan, London.

Knight, M. and Field, D. (1981) A silent conspiracy: coping with dying cancer patients on an acute surgical ward. *Journal of Advanced Nursing*, **6**, 221–269.

Kobasa, S.C., Hilker, R.R.J. and Maddi, S.R. (1979) Who stays healthy under stress? *Journal of Occupational Medicine*, **21**, 595–598.

Kovacs, M. and Beck, A.T. (1978) Maladaptive cognitive structures and depression. *American Journal of Psychiatry*, **135**, 525–533.

Kubler-Ross, E. (1970) *On Death and Dying*, Tavistock, London.

Kubler-Ross, E. (1986) *Death: The Final Stage of Growth*, Prentice Hall, Englewood Cliffs, NJ.

Kurpius, D.J., Baker, R.D. and Thomas, I.D. (1977) *Supervision of Applied Training*, Greenwood Press, New York.

Lanceley, A. (1985) Use of controlling language in the rehabilitation of the elderly. *Journal of Advanced Nursing*, **10**, 125–135.

Lange, A. and Jakubowski, P. (1978) *The Assertive Option: Your Rights and Responsibilities*, Research Press, Champaign, IL.

Lazarus, R.L. (1966) *Psychological Stress and the Coping Process*, McGraw Hill, New York.

Lazarus, R.S. and Folkman, S. (1984) *Stress, Appraisal and Coping*, Springer, New York.

Leavitt, H.J. (1951) Some effects of certain communication patterns on group performance. *Journal of Abnormal and Social Psychology*, **46**, 38–50.

Lendrum, S. and Symes, G, (1992) *The Gift of Tears: A Practical Approach to Loss and Bereavement Counselling*, Routledge, London.

Lewin, K. (1951) *Field Theory in Social Science*, Harper, New York.

Lewis, S. and Cooper, C.L. (1989) *Career Couples: Contemporary Lifestyles and How to Manage Them*, Unwin Hyman, London.

Ley, P. (1972) Primacy, rated importance and recall of medical information. *Journal of Health and Social Behaviour*, **13**, 311–317.

Ley, P. (1989) Improving patients' understanding, recall, satisfaction and compliance, in *Health Psychology: Process and Applications*, (ed. A. Broome), Chapman & Hall, London.

Leyens, J.-P. and Codol, J.-P. (1988) Social cognition, in *Introduction to Social Psychology*, (eds M. Hewstone, W. Stroebe, J.-P. Codol and G.M. Stephenson), Blackwell, Oxford.

Lillie, F. (1985) The wider social context of interpersonal skills in nursing, in *Interpersonal Skills in Nursing: Research and Applications*, (ed. C. Kagan), Croom Helm, London.

Lindenfield, G. (1986) *Assert Yourself*, Thorsens, Wellingborough, Northamptonshire.

Lindop, E. (1989) Individual stress and its relationship to termination of nurse training. *Nurse Education Today*, **9**, 172–179.

Llewelyn, S. (1984) The cost of giving: emotional growth and emotional stress, in *Understanding Nurses*, (ed. S. Skevington), John Wiley, Chichester.

Llewelyn, S.P. (1989) Caring: the costs to nurses and relatives, in *Health Psychology: Process and Applications*, (ed. A. Broome), Chapman & Hall, London.

Long, L., Paradise, L. and Long, T. (1981) *Questioning: Skills for the Helping Process*, Brookes/Cole, Monterey, CA.

Looker, T. and Gregson, O. (1989) *Stresswise*, Hodder & Stoughton, London.

Lorensen, M. (1983) Effects of touch on patients during a crisis situation in hospital, in *Nursing Research: Ten Studies in Patient Care*, (ed. J. Wilson-Barnett), John Wiley, Chichester.

Lorenz, K. (1963) *On Aggression*, Methuen, London.

Luft, J. (1969) *Of Human Interaction*, National Press Books, Palo Alto, CA.

Lukes, S. (1974) *Power: A Radical View*, Macmillan, London.

McCann, S.A. and McKenna, H.P. (1993) An examination of touch between nurses and elderly patients in a continuing care setting in Northern Ireland. *Journal of Advanced Nursing*, **18**(5), 838–846.

McConnell, E.A. (1982) *Burnout in the Nursing Profession: Coping Strategies, Causes and Costs*, C.V. Mosby, St Louis, MO.

McCrane, E., Lambert, V.A. and Lambert, C.E. (1987) Work stress, hardiness and burnout among hospital staff nurses. *Nursing Research*, **36**, 374–380.

McGuire, W.J. (1981) Theoretical foundations of campaigns, in *Public Communication Campaigns*, (eds R.E. Rice and W.J. Paisley), Sage Publications, Beverly Hills, CA.

Macleod-Clark, J. (1983) Nurse–patient communication: an analysis of conversations from surgical wards, in *Nursing Research: Ten Studies in Patient Care*, (ed. J. Wilson-Barnett), John Wiley, Chichester.

Macleod-Clark, J. (1984) Verbal communication in nursing, in *Recent Advances in Nursing 7: Communication* (ed. A. Faulkner), Churchill Livingstone, Edinburgh.

Macleod-Clark, J., Hopper, L. and Jesson, A. (1991) Progression to counselling. *Nursing Times*, **87**, 41–43.

Maddi, S.R. and Kobasa, S.C. (1984) *The Hardy Executive: Health Under Stress* Dow Jones–Irwin, Homewood, IL.

Maddux, R.B. (1988) *Team Building: An Exercise in Leadership*, Kogan Page, London.

Maguire, P. (1985) Deficiences in key interpersonal skills, in *Interpersonal Skills in Nursing: Research and Applications*, (ed. C. Kagan), Croom Helm, London.

Markus, H. and Zajonc, R.B. (1985) The cognitive perspective in social psychology, in *Handbook of Social Psychology*, (eds G.Lindzey and E. Aronson), Random House, New York.

Marsella, A.J., DeVos, G. and Hsu, F.L.K. (eds) (1985) *Culture and Self: Asian and Western Perspectives*, Tavistock, New York.

Marsh, P., Rosser, E. and Harré, R. (1978) *The Rules of Disorder*, Routledge & Kegan Paul, London.

Marshall, J. (1980) Stress amongst nurses, in *White Collar and Professional Stress*, (ed. C. Cooper and J. Marshall), John Wiley, Chichester.

Marshfield, G. (1985) Issues arising from teaching interpersonal skills in general nursing, in *Interpersonal Skills in Nursing: Research and Applications*, (ed. C. Kagan), Croom Helm, London.

Marteau, T.M. (1989) Health beliefs and attributions, in *Health Psychology: Process and Applications*, (ed. A. Broome), Chapman & Hall, London.

Maslach, C. (1982) *Burned Out: The Costs of Caring*, Prentice Hall, Englewood Cliffs, NJ.

Maslow, A.H. (1970) *Motivation and Personality*, 2nd edn, Harper & Row, New York.

Maslow, A.H. (1971) *The Farther Reaches of Human Nature*, Penguin, Harmondsworth, Middlesex.

Maynard, C.K. and Chitty, K.K. (1979) Dealing with anger: guidelines for nursing intervention. *Journal of Psychiatric Nursing and Mental Health Services*, **17**, 36–41.

Mayou, R. (1984) Sick role, illness behaviour and coping. *British Journal of Psychiatry*, **144**, 320–322.

Mead, G.H. (1934) *Mind, Self and Society*, University of Chicago Press, Chicago, IL.

Mechanic, D. (1986) The concept of illness behavior: culture, situation, and personal predisposition. *Psychological Medicine*, **16**, 1–7.

Menzies, I. (1960) A case study on the functioning of social systems as a defence against anxiety. A report of the nursing service in a general hospital. *Human Relations*, **Nov.**, 13–32.

Metcalfe, J. and Curtis, C. (1992) Feeding on support. *Community Care Inside*, **30 July**, vi–vii.

Milgram, S. (1974) *Obedience to Authority*, Harper & Row, New York.

Milne, D. and Watkins, F. (1986) An evaluation of the effects of shift rotation on nurses' stress, coping and strain. *International Journal of Nursing Studies* **23**, 139–146.

Morgan, G. (1986) *Images of Organization*, Sage Publications, London.

Morris, J. (1991) *Able Lives: Womens' Experiences of Paralysis*, Women's Press, London.

Moss, R.A. (1986) The role of learning history in current sick role behaviour and assertion. *Behaviour, Research and Therapy*, **24**, 681–683.

Mucchielli, R. (1972) *Face to Face in the Counselling Interview*, (trans. H. Hudson, 1983), Macmillan, London.

Mullender, A. and Ward, D. (1991) *Self-Directed Group Work: Users Taking Action for Empowerment*, Whiting & Birch, London.

Mullins, J. (1989) *Management and Organisational Behaviour*, 2nd edn, Pitman, London.

Murgatroyd, S. and Woolfe, R. (1982) *Coping with Crisis: Understanding and Helping People in Need*, Harper & Row, London.

Murphy, L. (1983) A comparison of relaxation methods for reducing stress in nursing personnel. *Human Factors*, **25**, 431.

National Health Service and Community Care Act 1990, HMSO, London.

Nattrass, H. (1992) Total quality management within a district, *Quality in Health Care: 1, Supplement: Raising Quality in the NHS*, BMJ Publications, London.

Nelson-Jones, R. (1983) *Practical Counselling Skills*, Holt, Rinehart & Winston, London.

Nelson-Jones, R. and Dryden, W. (1979) Anticipated risk and gain from negative and positive self-disclosure. *British Journal of Social and Clinical Psychology*, **18**, 79–80.

Nelson-Jones, R. and Strong, S.R. (1976) Positive and negative self-disclosures, timing and personal attraction. *British Journal of Social and Clinical Psychology*, **15**, 323–325.

Newman, O. (1972) *Defensible Space*, Architectural Press, London.

Nguyen, T.D., Heslin, R. and Nguyen, M.L. (1975) The meaning of touch: sex differences. *Journal of Communication*, **25**, 92–103.

Nicholls, J.R. (1985) A new approach to situational leadership. *Leadership and Organization Development Journal*, **6**, 2–7.

Nisbett, R.E. and Ross, L. (1980) *Human Inference: Strategies on Shortcomings in Social Judgement*, Prentice Hall, Englewood Cliffs, NJ.

Nisbett, R.E. and Schachter, S. (1966) Cognitive manipulation of pain. *Journal of Experimental Social Psychology*, **2**, 227–236.

Niven, N. (1989) *Health Psychology*, Churchill Livingstone, Edinburgh.

Owens, R.G. and Ashcroft, J.B. (1985) *Violence: A Guide for the Helping Professions*, Croom Helm, London.

Paine, W.S. (1982) *Job Stress and Burnout*, Sage Publications, Beverly Hills, CA.

Parker, I. and Burman, E. (eds) (1993) *Discourse Analytic Research: Repertoires and Readings of Texts in Action*, Routledge, London.

Parkes, K.R. (1980) Occupational stress amongst student nurses. *Nursing Times*, **76**, 113–119.

Parsons, T. (1951) *The Social System*, Free Press, New York.

Pearlin, L. and Schooler, C. (1978) The structure of coping. *Journal of Health and Social Behavior*, **19**, 2–21.

Pepler, C. J. and Lynch, A. (1991) Relational messages of control in nurse–patient interactions with terminally ill patients with AIDS and cancer. *Journal of Palliative Care*, **7**, 18–29.

Peterson, C. and Seligman, M.E.P. (1984) Causal explanations as a risk factor for depression: theory and evidence. *Psychological Review*, **91**, 347–374.

Peterson, M. (1988) The norms and values held by three groups of nurses concerning psychosocial nursing practice. *International Journal of Nursing Studies*, **25**, 85–105.

Petty, R.E. and Cacioppo, J.T. (1981) *Attitudes and Persuasion: Classic and Contemporary Approaches*, William C. Brown, Dubuque, IO.

Pfeffer, N. (1992) Strings attached. *Health Services Journal*, **2 April**, 22–23.

Pfeffer, N. and Coote, A. (1992) *Is Quality Good For You? A Critical Review of Quality Assurance in Welfare Services*, Institute for Public Policy Research, London.

Pfeiffer, J.W. and Jones, J.E. (1974) *A Handbook of Structured Experiences for Human Relations Training*, University Associates, La Jolla, CA.

Plant, R. (1987) *Managing Change and Making it Stick*, Fontana, London.

Pope, B. (1986) *Social Skills Training for Psychiatric Nurses*, Harper & Row, London.

Porritt, L. (1990) *Interaction Strategies: An Introduction for Health Professionals*, 2nd edn, Churchill Livingstone, Edinburgh.

Price, V.A. (1982) *Type A Behavior Pattern*, Academic Press, New York.

Proctor, B. (1988) *Supervision: A Working Alliance Videotape Training Manual*, Alexia Publications, St Leonards on Sea, Sussex.

Rakos, R.F. (1991) *Assertive Behaviour: Theory, Research and Training*, Routledge, London.

Rigge, M. and Cole, A. (1993) Involving patients and consumers. *Health Services Journal*, Management Guide.

Rijsman, J.B. (1983) The dynamics of social competition in personal and categorical comparison situations, in *Current Issues in European Social Psychology*, vol.1, (eds W. Doise and S. Moscovici), Cambridge University Press, Cambridge.

Roberts, D. (1984) Nonverbal communication, popular and unpopular patients, in *Recent Advances in Nursing 7: Communication* (ed. A. Faulkner), Churchill Livingstone, Edinburgh.

Robinson, E.J. (1989) Patients' contributions to the consultation, in *Health Psychology: Process and Applications*, (ed. A. Broome), Chapman & Hall, London.

Robinson, W.P. (1972) *Language and Social Behaviour*, Penguin, Harmondsworth, Middlesex.

Rogers, C.R. (1951) *Client Centred Therapy*, Constable, London.

Rogers, C.R. (1957) The necessary and sufficient conditions of therapeutic personality change. *Journal of Consulting Psychology*, **21**, 95–105.

Rogers, C.R. (1961) *On Becoming a Person*, Houghton Mifflin, Boston, MA.

Rogers, C.R. (1975) Empathic: an unappreciated way of being. *Counselling Psychologist*, **5**, 2–10.

Rogers, C.R. (1980) *A Way of Being*, Houghton Mifflin, Boston, MA.

Rogers, C.R. (1983) *Freedom to Learn for the Eighties*, Merrill, Columbus, OH.

Rokeach, M. (1968) *Beliefs, Attitudes and Values*, Jossey Bass, Beverley Hills, CA.

Rosenberg, M.J. and Hovland, C.I. (1960) Cognitive, affective and behavioral components of attitudes, in *Attitude Organisation and Change*, (eds C.I. Hovland and M.J. Rosenberg), Yale University Press, New Haven, CT.

Rosenstock, I.M. (1974) The health belief model and preventive health behavior. *Health Education Monographs*, **2**, 354–386.

Rosenstock, I.M. (1990) The health belief model: explaining health behavior through expectancies, in *Health Behavior and Health Education: Theory, Research and Practice*, (eds F.M. Lewis and B.K. Rimer), Jossey Bass, San Francisco.

Rosenthal, P. and Jacobson, L. (1968) *Pygmalion in the Classroom: Teacher Expectation and Pupils' Intellectual Development*, Holt, Rinehart & Winston, New York.

Rowe, D. (1983) *Depression: The Way Out of Your Prison*, Routledge & Kegan Paul, London.

Schachter, S. and Singer, J. (1962) Cognitive, social and physiological determinants of emotional state. *Psychological Review*, **69**, 378–399.

Schmidt, D. (1973) Supervision: a sharing process. *Child Welfare*, **41**, 436–446.

Schmidt, W.H. (1974) Conflict: A powerful process for (good or bad) change. *Management Review*, **63**, 4–10.

Scott, J. and Rochester, A. (1984) *Effective Management Skills: Managing People*, Sphere, London.

Seligman, M.E.P. (1975) *Helplessness: On Depression, Development and Death*, Freeman, San Francisco.

Selye, H. (1956) *The Stress of Life*, McGraw Hill, New York.

Selye, H. (1980) The stress concept today, in *Handbook on Stress and Anxiety*, (eds I.L. Kutash, L.B. Schlesinger *et al.*), Jossey Bass, San Francisco, CA.

Shaw, M.E. (1981) *Group Dynamics: The Social Psychology of Small Group Behavior*, 3rd edn, McGraw Hill, New York.

Smith, M.J. (1975) *When I say No I Feel Guilty*, Bantam, London.

Smith, P. (1992) *The Emotional Labour of Nursing (How Nurses Care)*, Macmillan, London.

Snyder, M. (1987) *Public Appearances and Private Realities: The Psychology of Self-Monitoring*, Freeman, New York.

Spurgeon, P. and Barwell, F. (1991) *Implementing Change in the NHS: A Practical Guide for General Managers*, Chapman & Hall/HSMC, London.

Stahlberg, D. and Frey, D. (1988) Attitudes I: structure, measurement and functions, in *Introduction to Social Psychology*, (eds M. Hewstone, W. Stroebe, J.-P. Codol and G.M. Stephenson), Blackwell, Oxford.

Stamp, G. (1992) *One Year On: The Nurse Executive Director Post*. NHS Management Executive, London.

Steiner, C. (1981) *The Other Side of Power*, Grove Press, New York.

Steptoe, A. (1991) Psychological coping, individual differences and physiological stress response, in *Personality and Stress: Individual Differences in the Stress Response*, (eds C. Cooper and R. Paine), John Wiley, Chichester.

Stewart, W. (1975) Nursing and counselling: a conflict of roles? *Nursing Mirror*, **140**, 71–73.

Stewart, W. (1983) *Counselling in Nursing: A Problem Solving Approach*, Harper & Row, London.

Stockwell, F. (1972) *The Unpopular Patient*, Royal College of Nursing, London (republished by Croom Helm, 1984).

Stone, G. and Farberman, H. (1970) *Social Psychology Through Symbolic Interaction*, Xerox College Publishing, Waltham, MA.

Stroebe, W. and Jonas, K. (1988) Attitudes II: strategies of attitude change, in *Introduction to Social Psychology*, (eds M. Hewstone, W. Stroebe, J.-P. Codol and G.M. Stephenson), Blackwell, Oxford.

Strongman, K. (1979) *Psychology for the Paramedical Professions*, Croom Helm, London.

Sutherland, V. and Cooper, C.L. (1990) *Understanding Stress*, Chapman & Hall, London.

Tait, A. (1985) Issues arising from mastectomy nursing, in *Interpersonal Skills in Nursing: Research and Applications*, (ed. C. Kagan), Croom Helm, London.

Tajfel, H. (1978) *Differentiation Between Social Groups: Studies in the Psychology of Intergroup Relations*, Academic Press, London.

Tajfel, H. (ed.) (1982a) *Social Identity and Intergroup Relations*, Cambridge University Press, Cambridge.

Tajfel, H. (1982b) Social psychology of intergroup relations. *Annual Review of Psychology*, **33**, 1–30.

Taylor, D. (1989) Citizenship and social power. *Critical Social Policy*, **26**, 19–31.

Thompson, C. (ed.) (1991) *Changing the Balance: Power and People Who Use Services*, Community Care Project, NCVO, London.

Thompson, D.R., Webster, R.A. and Meddis, R. (1990) In hospital counselling for first-time myocardial infarction patients and spouses: effects on satisfaction. *Journal of Advanced Nursing*, **15**, 1064–1069.

Totman, R. (1979) *Social Causes of Illness*, Souvenir Press, London.

Trower, P. (ed.) (1984) *Radical Approaches to Social Skills Training*, Croom Helm, London.

Trower, P., Bryant, B. and Argyle, M. (1978) *Social Skills and Mental Health*, Methuen, London.

Truax, C.B. and Carkhuff, R.R. (1967) *Towards Effective Counselling and Psychotherapy*, Aldine Press, Chicago, IL.

Tuckman, B.W. (1965) Development Sequence in Small Groups. *Psychological Bulletin*, **63**, 384–99.

Turner, J. and Giles, H. (eds) (1981) *Intergroup Behaviour*, Blackwell, Oxford.

Vachon, M.L.S. and Lyall, W.A.C. (1976) Applying psychiatric techniques to management of stress in health professionals working with advanced cancer patients. *Death Education*, **1**, 365–375.

Valins, S. (1972) Persistent effects of information about internal reactions, in *The Cognitive Alteration of Feeling States*, (eds H. London and R.A. Nisbett), Aldine Press, Chicago, IL.

Vaughan, B. and Pillmoor, M. (1989) *Managing Nursing Work*, Scutari, London.

von Cranach, M. and Harre, R. (1982) *The Analysis of Action: Recent Theoretical and Empirical Advances*, Cambridge University Press, Cambridge.

Walsh, M. and Ford, P. (1989) *Nursing Rituals, Research and Rational Actions*, Heinemann, London.

Ward, M. (1988) Sociolinguistics and the nursing process. *Senior Nurse*, **8**(11), 21–23.

Wegner, D.M. and Vallacher, R.R. (1977) *Implicit Personality: An Introduction to Social Cognition*, Oxford University Press, New York.

Weinberger, M., Hiner, S.L. and Tierney, W.M. (1987) In support of hassels as a measure of stress in predicting health outcomes. *Journal of Behavioural Medicine*, **10**, 19–31.

White, J.A. (1988) Touching with intent: therapeutic massage. *Holistic Nursing Practice*, **2**, 63–67.

Whittaker, D.S. (1985) *Using Groups to Help People*, Routledge & Kegan Paul, London.

Wilkinson, S. (1991) Factors which influence how nurses communicate with cancer patients. *Journal of Advanced Nursing*, **16**, 677–688.

Wilmott, M. (1989) The sick role and related concepts, in *Health Psychology: Process and Applications*, (ed. A. Broome), Chapman & Hall, London.

Wilson Barnett, J. (1981) Communicating with patients in general wards, in *Communication in Nursing Care*, (eds W. Bridge and J. Macleod Clark), HM & M , London.

Winn, L. (ed.) (1990) *Power to the People – The Way to Responsive Services in Health and Social Care*, King's Fund Centre, London.

Worchel, S. and Brehm, J.W. (1971) Direct and implied social restoration of freedom. *Journal of Personality and Social Psychology*, **18**, 294–304.

Wortman, C.B. and Brehm, J. (1975) Responses to uncontrollable outcomes: an integration of reactance theory and the learned helplessness model. *Advances in Experimental Social Psychology*, **8**, 278–336.

Wright, H. (1991) The patient, the nurse, his life and her mother: psycho-dynamic influences in nurse education and practice. *Psychoanalytic Psycho-therapy*, **5**, 139–149.

Wright, S. (1990) *My Patient, My Nurse: A Guide to Primary Nursing*, Scutari, London.

Yasko, J.M. (1983) Variables which predict burnout experienced by oncology clinical nurse specialists. *Cancer Nursing*, **6**, 109–116.

Further reading

Abrams, D. and Hogg, M. (eds) (1990) *Social Identity Theory: Constructive and Critical Advances,* Harvester Wheatsheaf, Brighton.

Alban Metcalf, B. (1984) Microskills of leadership: a detailed analysis of managers in the appraisal interview, in *Leaders and Managers: International Perspectives on Managerial Behavior and Leadership,* (eds J.G. Hunt, D. Hosking, C.A. Schriesheim and R. Stewart), Pergamon Press, New York.

Argyle, M. (1988) *Bodily Communication,* 2nd edn, Methuen, London.

Arnold, E. and Bogg, K. (1989) *Interpersonal Relationships: Professional Communication Skills for Nurses,* W.B. Saunders, London.

Atkinson, G.G.M. (1977) *The Effective Negotiator: A Practical Guide to the Strategies and Tactics of Conflict Bargaining,* 2nd edn, Quest Research Publications, London.

Bandura, A. (1973) *Aggression: A Social Learning Analysis,* Prentice Hall, Englewood Cliffs, NJ.

Birkitt, I. (1991) *Social Selves,* Sage Publications, London.

Bond, M. (1988) Assertiveness training 1–8. *Nursing Times,* **84**, 9–16.

Brennan, A (1993) Preceptorship: Is it a workable concept? *Nursing Standard,* **7**(52), 34–36.

Briggs, K. (1986) Assertiveness: speak your mind. *Nursing Times,* **82**(26), 24–26.

Bundy, C. (1989) Cardiac disorders, in *Health Psychology: Process and Applications,* (ed. A. Broome), Chapman & Hall, London.

Constable, J.F. and Russell, D.W. (1986) The effects of social support and the work environment upon burnout among nurses. *Journal of Human Stress,* **12**, 20–26.

Davitz, J.R. (1964) *The Communication of Emotional Meaning,* McGraw Hill, New York.

Dohrenwend, B.S. and Dohrenwend, B.P. (eds) (1984) *Stressful Life Events and their Contexts,* Rutgers University Press, New Brunswick, NJ.

Dunham, R.G. and Brower, H.T. (1984) The effects of assertiveness training on the non-traditional role assumptions of geriatric nurse practitioners. *Sex Roles,* **11**, 911–921.

Egerton, R.B. (1967) *The Cloak of Competence: Stigma in the Lives of the Mentally Retarded,* University of California Press, Berkeley, CA.

Fink, S.C., Beak, J. and Taddeo, K. (1971) Organizational crisis and change. *Journal of Applied Behavioral Science,* **17**, 14–37.

Gergen, K.J. (1971) *The Concept of Self,* Holt, Rinehart & Winston, New York.

Gergen, K.J. (1977) The social construction of self knowledge. In *The Self: Psychological and Philosophical Issues,* (ed. T. Mischel), Rowman & Littlefield, Totowa, NJ.

Hargie, O. and McCartan, P.J. (1990) Assessing assertive behaviour of student nurses: a comparison of assertion measures. *Journal of Advanced Nursing,* **15**, 1370–1376.

HMSO (1989) Caring for People: Community Care in the Next Decade and Beyond, *Cm849*, HMSO, London.

Hormuth, S.E. (1984) Restructuring the ecology of the self: a model for self-concept change. Paper presented to the International Conference on Self and Identity, University College, Cardiff.

Hurst, K. (1993) *Problem Solving in Nursing Practice*, Scutari, London.

Kinney, C.D. (1985) A re-examination of nursing role conceptions. *Nursing Research*, **34**, 170–176.

Klein, R. (1985) Management in health care: the politics of innovation. *International Journal of Health Planning and Management*, **1**, 57–63.

Kleinke, C.L. (1986) *Meeting and Understanding People*, Freeman, New York.

Lally, J. (1988) When anger is a cry for help. *Community Living*, **July**, 16.

Lythe-Menzies, I. (1988) *Containing Anxiety in Institutions: Selected Essays*, Free Association Books, London.

McIntyre, T.J., Jeffrey, D.B. and McIntyre, S.L. (1984) Assertion training: the effectiveness of a comprehensive cognitive–behavioural treatment package with professional nurses. *Behaviour Research and Therapy*, **22**, 311–318.

May, C. (1990) Research on nurse–patient relationships: problems of theory, problems of practice. *Journal of Advanced Nursing*, **15**, 307–315.

Michelson, L., Molcan, K. and Poorman, S. (1986) Development and psychometric properties of the nurses' assertiveness inventory (NAI). *Behaviour Research and Therapy*, **24**, 77–81.

Numerof, R.E. (1978) Assertiveness training for nurses in a general hospital. *Health and Social Work*, **3**, 79–102.

O'Leary, A. (1985) Self efficacy and health. *Behaviour, Research and Therapy*, **23**, 437–451.

Parkes, C.M. (1971) *Bereavement: Studies of Grief in Adult Life*, Tavistock, London.

Salvage, J. (1985) *The Politics of Nursing*, Heineman, London.

Schlenker, B.R. (1985) *The Self and Social Life* McGraw Hill, New York.

Sue, S. and Zane, N. (1977) Learned helplessness: theory and community psychology, in *Community Psychology*, (eds M. Gibbs, J.R. Lachenmeyer and J.R. Sigal), Gardner Press, New York.

Suls, J. (1982) *Psychological Perspectives on the Self*, vol. 1, Lawrence Erlbaum Associates, Hillsdale, NJ.

Suls, J. and Greenwald, A.G. (1983) *Psychological Perspectives on the Self*, vol. 2 Lawrence Erlbaum Associates, Hillsdale, NJ.

Tajfel, H. (1981) *Human Groups and Social Categories: Studies in Social Psychology*, Cambridge University Press, Cambridge.

Tessey, C. (1988) Communication difficulties and assertive/negotiation skills. *Nursing*, **3**, 1002–1005.

White, I., Devenney, M., Bhaduri, R. *et al.* (1988) *Hearing the Voice of the Consumer*, Policy Studies Institute, London.

Index

Page numbers in **bold** refer to figures and page numbers in *italic* type refer to tables